The Reorganised National Health Service

THIRD EDITION, COMPLETELY REVISED

RUTH LEVITT and ANDREW WALL

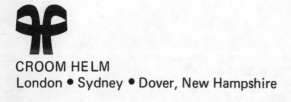

CROOM HELM
London • Sydney • Dover, New Hampshire

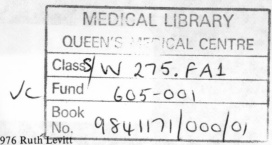
© 1976 Ruth Levitt
Revised material © 1984 Ruth Levitt and Andrew Wall
First published 1976
Revised and reprinted July 1976
Second edition 1977
Revised and reprinted 1979
Third edition 1984

Croom Helm Ltd, Provident House, Burrell Row,
Beckenham, Kent BR3 1AT

Croom Helm Australia Pty Ltd, First Floor,
139 King Street, Sydney, NSW 2001, Australia

British Library Cataloguing in Publication Data

Levitt, Ruth, 1950–
    — 3rd ed., completely rev.
    1. Medical care — England 2. Great
    Britain — National Health Service
    I. Title II. Wall, Andrew
    362.1'0942   RA395.G6

    ISBN 0–7099–1673–6
    ISBN 0–7099–1674–4 Pbk

Croom Helm, 51 Washington Street, Dover,
New Hampshire 03820, USA

Library of Congress Cataloging in Publication Data

Levitt, Ruth, 1950–
    The reorganised National Health Service.

    Bibliography: p.
    Includes index.
    1. Great Britain — National Health Service.
I. Wall, Andrew. II. Title.   DNLM: 1. State Medicine —
Great Britain. W275 FA1 L56r
RA412.5.G7L48   1984   362.1'0941   84–12745
ISBN 0–7099–1673–6
ISBN 0–7099–1674–4 (pbk.)

Typeset by Mayhew Typesetting, Bristol, UK
Printed and bound in Great Britain

CONTENTS

Contents

FIGURES

LIST OF ABBREVIATIONS

AHA	Area Health Authority
AHA(T)	Area Health Authority (Teaching)
ATO	Area Team of Officers
BMA	British Medical Association
BoG	Board of Governors
CHC	Community Health Council
CPSM	Council for Professions Supplementary to Medicine
DCP	District Community Physician
DHA	District Health Authority
DHSS	Department of Health and Social Security
DMC	District Medical Committee
DMT	District Management Team
DPT	District Planning Team
ENB	English National Board of the UKCC
FPC	Family Practitioner Committee
GMC	General Medical Council
GNC	General Nursing Council
GNP	Gross National Product
GP	General Practitioner
HAS	Health Advisory Service
HCPT	Health Care Planning Team
HMC	Hospital Management Committee
JCC	Joint Consultative Committee
JCPT	Joint Care Planning Team
LHC	Local Health Council
LMC	Local Medical Committee
MPC	Medical Practices Committee
NHS	National Health Service
PESC	Public Expenditure Survey Committee
RAWP	Resource Allocation Working Party
RHA	Regional Health Authority
RHB	Regional Hospital Board
RTO	Regional Team of Officers
SHHD	Scottish Home and Health Department
UKCC	United Kingdom Central Council for Nursing, Midwifery and Health Visiting
VPRS	Voluntary Price Regulation Scheme
WHTSO	Welsh Health Technical Services Organisation

MINISTERS OF HEALTH AND SECRETARIES OF STATE FOR SOCIAL SERVICES

Ministers of Health

1919–21	Dr. Christopher Addison
1921–22	Sir Alfred Mond
1922–23	Sir Arthur Griffith-Boscawen
1923	Neville Chamberlain
1923–24	Sir William Joynson-Hicks
1924	John Wheatley
1924–29	Neville Chamberlain
1929–31	Arthur Greenwood
1931	Neville Chamberlain
1931–35	Sir E. Hilton-Young
1935–38	Sir Kingsley Wood
1938–40	Walter Elliot
1940–41	Malcolm MacDonald
1941–43	Ernest Brown
1943–45	Henry Willink
1945–51	Aneurin Bevan
1951	Hilary Marquand
1951–52	Harry Crookshank
1952–55	Ian MacLeod
1955–57	Robin Turton
1957	Dennis Vosper
1957–60	Derek Walker-Smith
1960–63	Enoch Powell
1963–64	Anthony Barber
1964–68	Kenneth Robinson

Secretaries of State for Social Services

1968–70	Richard Crossman
1970–74	Sir Keith Joseph
1974–76	Barbara Castle
1976–79	David Ennals
1979–81	Patrick Jenkin
1981–	Norman Fowler

PREFACE

The National Health Service is a magnificent feature of the United Kingdom's post-war landscape. Not only has it provided employment and health care for millions of people, it has also enabled the whole society to take part in a generous system of distributing welfare more fairly. But despite undeniable and admirable achievements since its creation in 1946 the National Health Service has fallen short of the ambitious hopes of its founders in several significant ways.

It has neglected to pay adequate attention to ways of preventing disease and instead has concentrated on treating established ill-health. It has allowed resources to be chanelled disproportionately towards short-term hospital care at the expense of those needing long-term support both in hospital and the community. And it has not troubled to evaluate systematically the worth of procedures and treatments even though there has been a decline in the real growth of its resources.

Nevertheless the NHS continues to achieve a very great deal and efforts are continuously being made to improve its effectiveness. Most aspects of the NHS have been scrutinised and many policies have been modified. Some reforms arise from public and professional influences. Others reflect the essentially political foundations on which the NHS rests.

This books attempts to chart fully the evolution of the NHS from its creation to the present day. The major reorganisations of 1974 and 1982 are discussed in detail. The text has been written in the context of further reforms which are yet to be clarified and analysed. The book is a completely newly written account of the NHS which should be of interest to observers and participants alike. Since the original edition was published in 1976 much has altered, so only a few historical sections have been brought in from there. All the rest is new and could not have been written without help from a number of people. In particular we would like to thank John Palmer, Stephen Howard, Dora Frost and Robin Gourlay very warmly. Our special thanks go to Andy Penzato who has typed and retyped with outstanding dedication and good humour. We are, of course, responsible for errors and omissions. The permission of the Controller of Her Majesty's Stationary Office is acknowledged for the use of Crown Copyright material.

Ruth Levitt
Andrew Wall

1 BACKGROUND TO TODAY'S NATIONAL HEALTH SERVICE

This first chapter explores the first period of the NHS, looking at certain key events of the previous hundred years which provide important clues about why the NHS was originally created in its particular form and why it was the subject of two reorganisations within eight years. The basic elements of the NHS are the hospital services, the community-based services and the family practitioner services. Their separate origins will be traced to 1948 when the NHS began and will be followed through subsequent developments which culminated in the 1982 reorganisation.

Health Services Before 1948

Developments up to 1870

The concept of public responsibility for the health of individuals can be traced back at least as far as 1834 when the Poor Law Amendment Act was passed. This established that the parish workhouses should have sick wards where the able-bodied inmates could be treated when they became ill. However, the health of the community had long been neglected, and it became necessary for the workhouses to admit sick paupers living in the parish to their wards, since so many were dying in their homes, being unable to obtain any medical care for themselves. By 1848 the demand for institutional care was so great that the sick wards had become entirely devoted to sick paupers. The Public Health Act of that year acknowledged for the first time the State's responsibility in this matter through its creation of a central organising body called the General Board of Health. It was only able to achieve very few reforms because it did not possess the powers necessary to counter the vested interests of the Boards of Guardians, who were the local managers of the institutions concerned.

By 1851 the first links between workhouses and the voluntary hospitals were beginning to be forged. The origins of this second group of hospitals represented a complete contrast to the workhouses. They emerged from the philanthropy and altruism of the well-to-do, and the moral obligations of religious and charitable bodies, whereas the workhouses had developed in the eighteenth century to cope with

1

the problems of poverty and destitution. The voluntary hospitals were built and financed through donations and subscriptions and attracted the services of skilled doctors who, acting on their social conscience, treated the patients often without payment. These hospitals became selective in their admissions, leaving all but acute cases to be dealt with by the workhouses. The workhouses themselves sometimes subscribed to nearby voluntary hospitals so that they could transfer their more complicated and acute cases to them. In this way, ill-health became divided to mirror the social status of the two types of hospitals, but the load was not evenly shared – in 1861 there were estimated to be 50,000 sick paupers in the workhouses and 11,000 patients in the voluntary hospitals. The Metropolitan Poor Act of 1867 represents a further landmark in health care provision as it obliged local authorities within London to provide separate institutional care for tuberculosis, smallpox, fevers and insanity. One year later, another Poor Law Amendment Act established the same provision in the provinces.

Developments from 1870 to 1919

By the 1870s, the workhouses, isolation hospitals and asylums together with the voluntary hospitals could be described as a public service through which people had access to hospital care when they became ill. Conditions were often appalling by modern standards, and medicine had few effective tools for alleviating disease; most of the activity involved care rather than treatment, and care that was sometimes harshly and unwillingly distributed. It is possible that the stimulus to alter this inadequate state of affairs only came after the experience of war – particularly the Crimean and Boer wars – in which thousands of British soldiers died from disease. For every death from combat in Southern Africa there were at least four from typhoid and other fevers. The Army's Committee on Physical Deterioration reported that 48 per cent of recruits had to be rejected on physical grounds alone. Its recommendations were the basis for the establishment of the School Medical Service in 1907. In addition, the beginning of the twentieth century saw a new era in effective medical care with discoveries that put diagnostic, therapeutic and pathological efforts on a much more scientific footing. It was clear that the nineteenth-century hospitals could not ensure a healthy fighting force were there to be another war, so interest moved for the first time towards preventive methods of health care. But this did not happen rapidly for it depended on having general practitioners who could deal with the huge unmet demand for health education and care in the community.

In comparison with famous specialists in the voluntary hospitals who were able to build up large private practices, the general practitioners in the parishes derived much of their income from the capitation fees paid to them on contract by the friendly societies, trade unions and similar associations, in return for the provision of treatment and medicines to the members. Most of the wage-earning population, including a large proportion of the middle class, received their medical care in this way, through the payment of a flat rate contribution to their association. The benefits were only available to the wage earner himself — wives, children, the old and the disabled had to rely on out-patient departments and dispensaries of the voluntary hospitals or go without. In 1911, through the British Medical Association, the doctors put pressure on Lloyd George to protect their interests and, with the passing of the National Health Insurance Act, they were successful in changing the administrative control of their work to new insurance committees, on which they were represented. The Act made lower paid workers compulsorily insured for the services of a general practitioner and fixed the fee that the doctor could receive for every person on his list. However, this still left the majority of the population without any improvements in their general practitioner services.

Some local authorities had achieved many advances in public and environmental health, but since they could not be compelled to provide many health services at all, substantial differences in the amount and quality of their provision emerged across the country. In 1905, the Minority Report of the Poor Law Commission came out strongly in favour of intervention by central government in tackling poverty and ill-health. The government chose to act indirectly, through the provision of old age pensions and unemployment benefits rather than improving the health care system itself. The Ministry of Reconstruction, which was set up towards the end of the First World War continued to approach this problem indirectly by proposing that a Ministry of Health should be established, to take on all the functions of the Local Government Board and the work of the National Health Insurance Commission.

Developments from 1919 to 1942

The new Ministry of Health was established in 1919 but it only devoted a small part of its time and efforts to health service administration since the duties transferred to it from the Local Government Board were so numerous. Nevertheless, a radical stimulus to the provision of a nationally organised, comprehensive health service was provided in the Dawson Report.[1] It recommended a number of objectives including domiciliary services from doctors, pharmacists and local health authority staff; primary health centres with beds for general practitioners, diagnostic facilities, outpatient clinics, dental, ancillary and community services; secondary health centres for specialist diagnosis and treatment; supplementary services for infectious and mental illnesses; teaching hospitals with medical schools; the promotion of research; standardised clinical records; the establishment of a single authority to administer all medical and allied services with medical representation and local medical committees. Although this report was published in 1920, it identified the issues which have been central to most of the subsequent debate on the organisation of the health services to the present day.

Then in 1926, the Royal Commission on National Health Insurance stated that the ultimate solution would lie in the direction of divorcing the medical service entirely from the insurance system, and reorganising it together with other public health activities as a service to be supplied from the general public funds. The need for greater coordination between the various parts of the system was only slowly and partially met, as for instance through the Local Government Act, 1929, which transferred to the local authorities all the responsibilities of the Poor Law Boards of Guardians, and additionally permitted them to provide the full range of hospital treatment. However, there was no compulsion, so great variations in standards existed. Some local authorities actively worked towards providing modern buildings with good equipment and the beginnings of specialist care, while others continued to have crowded, dark and understaffed wards in their old workhouse buildings.

The next important stimulus to reform in the scheme of health care did not come until 1939 when, as part of their wartime measures, the government set up the Emergency Medical Service. This made the Minister of Health responsible for the treatment of casualties, and thus enabled the central department to direct the day-to-day work of the voluntary and local authority hospitals for the first time. In return the government took over the financial burden of this provision, which until that time had been met by patients' contributions, local authority rates, and the funds of the voluntary hospitals. Many prefabricated buildings were erected to create more beds and to compensate for those destroyed by enemy bombings. Outpatient departments, operating theatres and X-ray departments were set up, and through the local cooperation of medical and administrative staff, a much more effective scheme of care began to develop. Special centres grew up to deal with specific types of injury, and the blood transfusion service became a nationally organised effort that could cope far better with the demands of the war emergency. This 'national hospital service' was very quickly formed without any statutory change in ownership or management and showed, for the first time, albeit under the pressure of war, what sort of developments could arise from central leadership and coordination. In 1941 Ernest Brown, the Minister of Health, announced that the government had commissioned an independent inquiry into the state of all the country's hospitals and their ability to provide adequate facilities. These hospital surveys confirmed clearly that there were great inequalities of provision, that many of the public's needs were not being properly met and, above all, that without thorough coordination of effort there would be insufficient improvement.[2] Although the findings were hardly disputed there was a considerable divergence of views on the best way to finance the necessary reforms, and on the question of whether central government should assume ownership and control of the existing hospitals.

The Creation of the National Health Service

In 1942 the Beveridge Report was published, and it made far-reaching recommendations that formed the basis for the postwar system of social welfare services.[3] But in addition it took as its central assumption the idea that a comprehensive system of health care was essential to any scheme for improving living standards. To Sir William Beveridge, the term 'comprehensive' meant medical treatment available for every citizen, both in the home and in hospital, provided by general practitioners, specialists, dentists and opticians, nurses and midwives, and the provision of surgical appliances and rehabilitation services. He thought these should be available to all citizens as and when they should need them.

The Coalition government announced in 1943 that it accepted the need for a comprehensive scheme of health care, and it started negotiations with a number of bodies. The first plan envisaged a unified health service with one administrative unit taking full responsibility for local provision. The units would be administered by regional local government or by joint local and health authorities. The hospitals would be partially taken into national ownership and general practitioners would

be full-time salaried servants. The British Medical Association was out-
raged at these proposals which it saw as originating from the influence
of the National Association of Local Government Officers, and the
Society of Medical Officers of Health, so it withdrew from the discussions and progress was temporarily halted. Later in 1943 Henry
Willink replaced Ernest Brown as Minister of Health and set about
devising a scheme that would be acceptable to the various interest
groups. In 1944 he published a White Paper, *A National Health
Service*,[4] which described a system of administration with the central
responsibility vested in the Ministry of Health, to be advised by an
appointed Central Health Services Council. Local organisations would
be based on joint local authority areas which would in turn be advised
by local versions of the Central Health Services Council. They would
take over the local authority hospitals and would determine the financial compensation to be paid for the voluntary hospitals boards' participation in the public scheme. General practitioners would be under
contract to a central medical board with local committees and would be
paid, as in the National Health Insurance system, on a per capita basis,
unless they worked from a health centre provided by the local
authority – in which case they would receive a salary. The central
board would be able to regulate the distribution of practices all over the
country. Although this plan failed to satisfy the varying interests,
several of its proposals were retained in the final legislation.

The government was indecisive, and discussions dragged on for
fifteen months until a revised version was drawn up. This differed from
the White Paper in proposing a two-tiered administrative structure in
the form of regional and local planning authorities, and in which ownership and administration of the hospitals was to remain with the local
authorities and voluntary hospital boards. Instead of the central
medical board of the White Paper, a series of local committees similar
to the existing local insurance committees of the National Health
Insurance system was proposed. This plan therefore dropped the idea
of joint administration of the hospital and local authority services
(which was not raised again until 1968), but it did establish the idea of
regional and local levels of management. It did not tackle the problem
of doctors' remuneration and the principle of health centre practice
was relegated to 'experimental' status. These last points have been of
continuing controversy in the health service, but in this case meant that
Willink had to drop the idea of a fully integrated service in order to
meet the negotiating demands of as many groups as possible.

Although the Labour Party conference of 1944 came out in favour

Figure 1 *The National Health Service 1948–74*

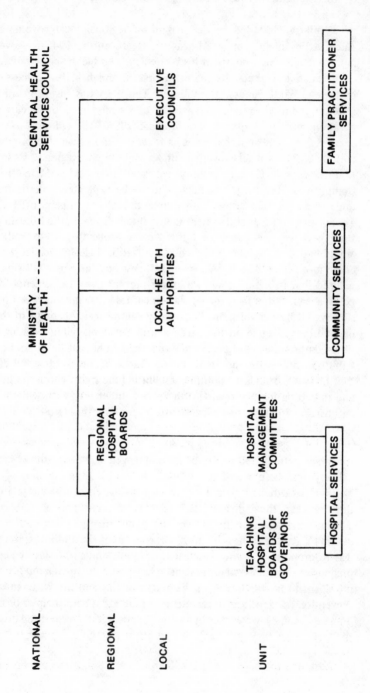

NATIONAL

REGIONAL

LOCAL

UNIT

MINISTRY OF HEALTH

CENTRAL HEALTH SERVICES COUNCIL

REGIONAL HOSPITAL BOARDS

TEACHING HOSPITAL BOARDS OF GOVERNORS

HOSPITAL MANAGEMENT COMMITTEES

LOCAL HEALTH AUTHORITIES

EXECUTIVE COUNCILS

HOSPITAL SERVICES

COMMUNITY SERVICES

FAMILY PRACTITIONER SERVICES

of a full-time salaried service based on regional local government, Aneurin Bevan did not, as Minister of Health in the 1945–51 government, include these points in his White Paper. In fact he adopted much of the detail worked out for earlier plans, and held few discussions before the White Paper was published. The BMA was suspicious of his intentions and organised a campaign of its members to boycott cooperation with the government. In March 1946 the *National Health Service Bill*[5] was published, and its main new point was the proposed nationalisation of all hospitals under appointed Regional Hospital Boards, with local responsibility delegated to Hospital Management Committees. Teaching hospitals were to be separately administered under Boards of Governors with a direct link to the Ministry of Health. There were however still a great many details to be worked out in the time between the passing of the Act in November 1946 and the 'appointed day', 5 July 1948, when the National Health Service would come into effect. The BMA resumed discussions early in 1947 since it realised that its action could no longer prevent the arrangements from going ahead, but in fact, the legislation ensured that the medical profession would have a voice on all statutory committees. Accounts of these negotiations disagree on the part Aneurin Bevan played in reaching the final compromises. Although some observers hold that he did not contribute many original points to the substance of the Act, it seems clear that he was particularly skilful in exploiting the splits within the BMA, and in getting the National Health Service under way with widespread enthusiasm amongst the staff and institutions concerned.

How the New National Health Service Worked

Although patients received broadly unchanged services at the point of delivery just before and just after 5 July 1948, the creation of the National Health Service did represent a radical change in the relationship between the individual citizen and the State, and it established a firm government commitment to developing and improving the country's system of health care. In the words of the 1946 Act, the aim was to promote '. . . the establishment in England and Wales of a comprehensive health service designed to secure improvement in the physical and mental health of the people of England and Wales and the prevention, diagnosis and treatment of illness'.[6] The principles of freedom and choice were upheld in that all people were entitled to use the service yet they still had the opportunity to go to doctors outside the service. Equally, doctors would have no interference in their clinical judgement and were free to take private patients while participating in the service. The achievement of the Act was to make benefits available to everyone free of charge, on the basis of need, thus ending the former restrictions of provision to those who were insured or those who could afford private treatment.

The Minister of Health was made personally responsible to Parliament for the provision of all hospital and specialist services on a national basis, and for the Public Health Laboratory Service, the Blood Transfusion Service and research concerned with the prevention, diagnosis and treatment of illness. He had indirect responsibility for the family practitioner and local authority health services. The Central Health Services Council and its professional Standing Advisory Committees were established to advise the Minister on the discharge of his duties, and to keep developments in the service under review. The fourteen Regional Hospital Boards (subsequently fifteen) were each focused on a university with a medical school, and teaching hospitals were separately administered by Boards of Governors. Hospital Management Committees were appointed to run the non-teaching hospitals on a day-to-day basis. The local health authorities were the county councils and the borough councils. Through their health committees they provided community and environmental health services including maternal and child welfare, health visiting, home nurses, vaccination and immunisation, care and after-care for mental illness and mental subnormality patients and the maintenance of health centres. Some of these had already been their responsibility before 1948 whilst others had been provided by a variety of other agencies. Executive Councils were established (usually to match the local health authorities) to administer the family practitioner services and received their finance directly from the Ministry of Health (see Figure 1). The Act also recognised the contribution that voluntary organisations could make in the field of health care by absorbing some of their activities into the NHS and giving financial aid to others operating outside the NHS. The school medical service continued to be run by the local education authorities and provided medical and dental inspections for children in state schools, and a child guidance service. The Industrial Health Service was organised by the Ministry of Labour mainly through the factory inspectorate. The armed forces retained their own health service quite separate from the NHS.

The Problems of the NHS

Just as the final form of the NHS in 1948 represented a compromise between the demands of several interest groups, so the problems that the service encountered between 1948 and 1974 were a reflection of the failure to meet the original hopes for a fully unified and comprehensive health service that had been expressed as far back as the beginning of the century. For example, when compulsory payments by patients were introduced for some parts of the service and when the weekly NHS contribution was established, the idea of a free service for all was breached. A more important problem was, however, that the demand for NHS care rose very rapidly and resources were often insufficient to be able to meet it. The uneven distribution of services that had existed before 1948 was not eradicated by the creation of the NHS, so many inequalities between regions were maintained. Because the administrative structure, with its bias towards hospital matters, had the strongest influence on policy-making in the central department, there was inadequate local liaison between hospital and community staff, with the result that services for the acutely ill tended to improve more rapidly while the needs of the chronically ill and disabled were comparatively neglected.

In 1953 the Minister of Health set up a committee to inquire into the costs of the NHS and its report, published three years later (the Guillebaud Report)[7] although acknowledging some deficiencies in the service, did not see structural alterations as a necessary measure at that time. One member of the committee, Sir John Maude, stated his reservations about this conservative position. He had identified for himself the weakness of the NHS as being its division into three parts operated by three sets of bodies having no organic connection with each other; their separate funding from central and local government sources underlined the weakness. The divisions caused preventive medicine, general practice and hospital practice to overlap, while the predominance of the hospital service had the effect of pushing general practice and social medicine into the background. Maude's view was that if local government administration and finance could be adequately reorganised then it might be possible to transfer the local responsibility of the NHS to them, thus arranging for a truly unified service.

The Beginnings of Reform

The first notable mention of a plan to unify the health service was made in the Porritt Report[8] which was compiled independently of the Ministry of Health by representatives of the medical profession. Its suggestion for local NHS administration under Area Health Boards, although not worked out in detail, at least indicated that the medical profession accepted in principle the need for unification. However, the Gillie Report (1963)[9] rejected unification of administration in favour of much greater efforts in developing the role of general practitioners. It suggested that family doctors alone could effectively coordinate the resources of hospital and community care on behalf of their patients, in relation to individual family and working conditions.

During this period, several other reports appeared and further Acts of Parliament were passed in relation to the NHS. They can be seen, in retrospect, to have reflected the problems being encountered in trying to overcome the deficiencies of the tripartite structure and represent tentative moves towards greater integration. The Cranbrook Report (1959)[10] for example was critical of the division between local authority and hospital maternity services. The Mental Health Act, 1959, radically altered the legislation on mental illness, reducing the grounds for compulsory admission and detention in mental hospitals. This coincided with the use of several new drugs leading to quicker and more effective psychiatric treatment which could more often be given on an outpatient basis. Mental hospitals began to discharge more patients back into the community and in 1961, Enoch Powell, the Minister of Health, predicted that half of these hospitals would be closed in ten years times. Although he was wrong in detail, progressively more mental hospital patients were transferred to community care.

In 1962, Powell published *A Hospital Plan for England and Wales*[11] which formulated the need for new hospitals in the light of projected population growth and the demand for hospital facilities in the coming ten years. It approved the development of district general hospitals for population units of about 125,000 people. The Bonham–Carter Report[12] on the functions of the district general hospital developed this concept in more detail, emphasising the need to plan hospital and community health services jointly. In 1967, the Salmon Report[13] published detailed recommendations for developing the senior nursing staff structure and the status of the profession in hospital management. The first report on the organisation of doctors in hospitals was published in 1967 (known as the Cogwheel Report)[14] and it proposed speciality groupings that would arrange clinical and administrative medical work more sensibly. These reports will be discussed in detail in later chapters, but are mentioned here to indicate the variety of efforts involved in trying to improve the tripartite structure. There was a growing acknowledgement of the complexity of the organisation and the corresponding need for effective management.

Preparation for Reorganisation

The necessity for a fundamental reorganisation of the service had not, however, become the subject of general discussion even though the administrative structure had remained unchanged for twenty years, and the various reports mentioned above had pointed out some of the serious faults that had arisen. The NHS was then composed of 15 Regional Hospital Boards, 36 Boards of Governors, 336 Hospital Management Committees, and 134 Executive Councils administering the services of 20,000 general practitioners while 175 local health authorities ran the community services.

The First Green Paper

The issue of reorganising these elements was first officially tackled on 6 November 1967 when Kenneth Robinson, the Minister of Health, stated in the House of Commons that he had begun a full and careful examination of the administrative structure of the NHS, not only in relation to the present, but looking twenty years ahead. He followed this in July 1968 with the publication of *The Administrative Structure of Medical and Related Services in England and Wales*,[15] now known as the First Green Paper. He took as his central theme the unification of health services in an area under one new body called the Area Board. This would replace the Regional Hospital Boards, Boards of Governors, Hospital Management Committees and Executive Councils, and take over certain functions previously held by the local health authorities. There would be forty to fifty Area Boards in direct contact with the Ministry of Health, and their boundaries would be related to those of local government, serving populations of between 750,000 and two to three millions.

These proposals were launched in anticipation of the reforms which might result from two inquiries which were being held at that time. The first was that of the Committee on Local Authority and Allied Personal Social Services (chaired by Frederick Seebohm)[16] which recommended, later in 1968, that all personal social services should be unified, including those administered by local authority health departments, in single new local authority departments with their own committee of elected representatives, and the appointment of directors of social services

trained in social work or social administration. The second was the
Royal Commission on Local Government in England,[17] whose report,
published in 1969, recommended the creation of new local authority
areas under unitary authorities, grouped into eight provinces each with
its own provincial council. The Commission's scheme aimed to loosen
the grip of central government over the control of planning and
management in local affairs through the communities' fuller participation in their public services. It saw the new unitary authorities as being
eminently suitable to take charge of the health services along the lines
suggested in the First Green Paper for ending the tripartite divisions,
but with the added advantage of being able to coordinate the health
services with the social services reorganised by the Seebohm proposals.
The significant stumbling block of finance was acknowleded by the
Commission – the cost of each authority's health services would be
far too great for the current rating system to bear – but it was hoped
that new sources of finance for local government would in any case be
worked out. The Layfield Committee's report on local government
finance[18] was not able to resolve this question. Of the three proposed
reforms, the First Green Paper, the Seebohm Report and the Royal
Commission's Report, only the Seebohm recommendations were
accepted, and the government implemented them in the Social Services
Act, 1970.

The Second Green Paper

In 1968, Richard Crossman succeeded Kenneth Robinson to become
the first Secretary of State for Social Servives in the new Department
of Health and Social Security. He published *The Future Structure of
the National Health Service*[19] known as the Second Green Paper, in
February 1970, which reflected some of the criticisms received about
the First Green Paper, as well as Crossman's own ideas. In it he stated
that the government had already decided on three important factors:
that the new health authorities would be independent of local government and directly responsible to the central department; that the public
health and personal social services would continue to be the responsibility of local government; that the boundaries of the new health
authorities would match those of local government. This second scheme
for the reorganisation suggested more health authorities than the first
attempt – ninety instead of forty or fifty, but it inserted Regional
Health Councils between them and the Department of Health and
Social Security (DHSS). These bodies were to take charge of hospital
and specialist planning. Crossman intended to publish a White Paper

that summer so that the Bills for health and local government reform could be put before Parliament early in 1972, permitting elections for the new local authorities[20] and appointments for the new health authorities to be completed in 1973 so that they could take over in 1974.

The Consultative Document

The General Election of June 1970 did not, however, return the Labour Party to power, so future plans for the health service awaited the decision of the new Conservative government's Secretary of State, Sir Keith Joseph. Almost one year later, in May 1971, he issued a Consultative Document[21] to interested parties only, without officially publishing it. Two months were allowed for comment so that the legislation could be prepared to come into force on 1 April 1974, the date already set by the local government reforms embodied in the Conservative White Paper, *Local Government in England*.[22] The Consultative Document rejected much of the Second Green Paper's plan but retained the proposal to incorporate local authority health services into the duties of the new area authorities, and to match health and local authorities' boundaries. Joseph's scheme brought hospitals, health centres and community nursing services under the new authorities; occupational health service provision was left with the Department of Employment and Productivity, but there was no decision on whether to take over the School Health Service from the Department of Education and Science. The major new feature was the proposal for a strong regional tier of authority to be responsible for planning, finance and building, with the power to direct the area authorities. Efficient management was the skill thought to be desirable amongst the membership of the authorities so professional representatives as such would not be necessary. The consumer's view would be voiced on Community Health Councils established outside the chain of authority. Social services would remain with the local authorities, and general practitioner services would be administered separately from the new authorities, retaining their distinct source of finance. Clinical teaching services would also be separate and organised on a regional basis. The Consultative Document also announced two 'expert studies' had been commissioned by the DHSS; Brunel University's Health Service Organisation Research Unit carried out work on the detailed management arrangements for the new authorities and their staff with particular emphasis on role relationships.[23] The management consultants McKinsey & Co. Inc. were also brought in to conduct trials with a few hospital management committees.

At the same time they advised on internal reorganisation at the DHSS itself.

Final Legislative Steps

The sequence of the final procedure to establish the reorganisation of the NHS involved publication of the Government's White Paper, *National Health Service Reorganisation: England*[24] in August 1972 followed by the *National Health Service Reorganisation Bill* in November 1972. After parliamentary debate, the National Health Service Reorganisation Act, 1973 was given Royal Assent on 5 July 1973 (i.e. exactly 25 years after the original 'appointed day').[25] The first phase of the investigations by the Study Group on the management arrangements was completed in February 1972, but the final report, *Management Arrangements for the Reorganised National Health Service*,[26] known as the Grey Book, did not appear until the end of 1972, after the White Paper had been published. The Working Party on Collaboration produced its first report in 1973. These reports contained the fruits of the Brunel and McKinsey studies. The DHSS started issuing a new series of circulars in 1972 to the existing health authorities and to members of the newly created 'shadow' authorities, detailing preparations for the reorganisation, and a news sheet called *NHS Reorganisation News*, but apart from these there was little information available and almost no public debate of the complicated issues involved. People working in the NHS began to realise that there would be a period of considerable uncertainty in relation to the jobs they might expect to obtain and the speed at which all the new appointments would be made. The National Health Service Staff Commission was appointed in 1972 to handle all the arrangements relating to recruitment and transfer of staff, and it was also made responsible for protecting the interests of staff under the new arrangements.

The publication of the Grey Book provided the skeleton of the new organisation, describing the Regional and Area Health Authorities, the District Management Teams, and outlining job descriptions for some of the new posts at all levels (see Figure 2). For those unfamiliar with the particular style of language that it employed, the Grey Book represented a puzzling basis on which to develop a grasp of the implications of the reorganisation. The main problem was also that preparations had to be made at speed in order to meet the deadline of 1 April 1974, and this discouraged thorough discussions of the impending changes. The Grey Book contained proposals which could be altered as a result of consultation, but the enforced haste transformed the

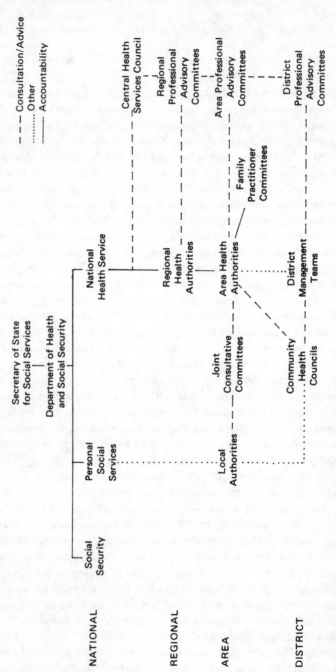

Figure 2 *The Reorganised National Health Service*

Source: Management Arrangements for the Reorganised National Health Service, HMSO, 1972

proposals into official edicts in the minds of many people. DHSS circular HRC(73) 3[27] in fact amended some of the Grey Book's statements, and the representations of certain professional groups against parts of the Grey Book continued to be discussed throughout 1974.

By June 1973 it had become clear that the programme of new staff appointments could not be completed by the following April, so the reorganised NHS would have to be launched with all but the most senior staff without formal contracts of employment. Although the need for a reorganisation of the NHS was hardly disputed and although this particular version of the reorganisation was widely supported, it is probably true that many staff working in the NHS and in outside, but related, bodies were not in a position to fully understand the thinking behind the preparations for 1974. The administrative arrangements were not as complete as the staff would have desired, but it is clear that their patients, as the focus of their efforts, were probably quite unaware that any reorganisation was taking place.

Yet on the very date at which the new NHS came into being, changes in its structure were already being planned. In February 1974 a Labour government replaced the Conservatives and the new administration was compelled to proceed with the reorganisation timed for the coming April even though the design was not of its making. The new Secretary of State, Barbara Castle, acknowledged the problems being encountered by the staff in implementing the reorganisation, but she was also determined to influence its development immediately. She set out her proposals in a consultative paper entitled *Democracy in the National Health Service*[28] and changes based on them were announced in July 1975.

Reasons for Creating the Area Health Authorities

In order to understand why it was thought necessary to establish a tier of authority at area level for the integrated administration of the NHS, it is helpful to return briefly to the criticisms that were being made about the NHS during the 1960s; the key arguments can be found in the Porritt Report, and the two Green Papers. The theme running through them was that despite its considerable achievements, the NHS was not organised in such as way that the three arms of the service could work efficiently and cooperatively. Without better dovetailing, satisfactory standards of patient care could not be assured because the poor liaison between hospitals, community services and general practitioners too often led to unacceptable delays and unnecessary suffering on the part of many patients.

The Medical Services Review Committee was appointed in the autumn of 1958 under the chairmanship of Sir Arthur Porritt with representatives from the Royal Colleges of Physicians, Surgeons, Obstetricians and Gynaecologists, the Society of Medical Officers of Health, the College of General Practitioners and the British Medical Association. Their report, published four years later, can reasonably be taken as the expression of the opinion of the medical profession at that time, and its unequivocal conclusion was that '. . . one administrative unit should become the focal point for all the medical services of an appropriate area, and that doctors and other personnel in all branches of the Service should be under contract with this one authority',[29] and that, '. . . the full advantages of the preventive and personal health services and their effective integration with the family doctor and hospital services can only be achieved by transferring both services and staff to the Area Health Boards'.[30]

But this view illustrates only part of what the NHS is intended to do. In fact it is not only concerned with the delivery of care to patients, but it is also required to allocate and reallocate resources, and these two functions are not the same – they are, rather, interdependent on each other. If the NHS was simply about the day-to-day treatment and prevention of illness, the arguments about a reorganisation would have focused on ensuring closer cooperation between all the staff involved in this activity. The additional emphasis given to 'management' of the services[31] indicates that it is also about planning for the future. The DHSS's internal reorganisation was intended to enable better planning and improved delegation of its authority to become possible.

In his foreword to the White Paper of 1972, the Secretary of State wrote of the reorganisation: 'It is about administration, not about treatment and care.'[32] The significance of the new authorities at area level now becomes clearer. The DHSS and the RHAs had to concentrate on strategic planning, whether nationally or regionally, while the Districts were concerned with the day-to-day delivery of health care. Only the Area Health Authorities were in a position to do some of both activities, and as such it may be helpful to regard them as having been the embodiment of an 'integrated' service. Put another way, if each part of the new structure had a clear precedent in the pre-1974 organisation, critics could have expressed the opinion that the reorganisation had simply given new names to all the old jobs and committees without really altering very much. But with the reorganisation, although many of its features were not wholly new, an exact ancestor of the Area Health Authorities is difficult to identify. In that sense, their existence could be said to have represented a focus for the hopes that the administrative rearrangement would prove to be a successful attempt to improve both the management and the delivery of health care.

Boundaries of the New Authorities

It must be remembered that the NHS reorganisation was planned in the context of the new arrangements for local authority personal social services and the reorganisation of local government. Both these reforms set down new geographical boundaries for their respective spheres of administration, facts which could not be ignored by the health service. Therefore another important element in the debate about the NHS was the administrative boundaries that the new area authorities would observe. The First Green Paper, which was published in advance of the report from the Royal Commission on Local Government, did not specify boundaries of the area authorities, but did entertain the possibility that health and local government could be jointly administered. However, the Second Green Paper favoured the separate administration of health services, but within the same geographical areas as were defined for local authorities.

The question is, what boundaries are most suitable for decentralised administration of the NHS: should they reflect the incidence of ill-health or should they conform to existing boundaries of complementary agencies? The answer depends on the previous point about whether the NHS administration is concerned with delivery of care to people or about strategic planning of its available resources. It would seem that if provision of services is the primary purpose, then organisation should take account of the distribution of relative prevalence of disease. However, if realistic planning is the aim, then conterminosity with local authority boundaries (i.e. identical boundaries) would be desirable. Few people would be happy to state a preference between these options, and the creation of Area Health Authorities with the same boundaries as local government, although emphasising the planning function, also underlined the recognition of the need for close collaboration between all parts of the health service and the staff of other agencies.[33]

Inequalities

Epidemiological studies have demonstrated that ill-health is associated with a number of social factors such that urban areas of declining employment with a high degree of overcrowding, low standards of housing and low wages are those with high mortality rates. Yet the pattern of health service provision has been a patchwork, essentially unrelated to population and mortality rates from particular diseases; this is partly what is meant by 'regional inequalities'. However, the difficulty of altering the balance of local services to handle local needs (which was the job of the Area Health Authorities) should not be underestimated. The historical pattern of distribution of resources and the comparative rigidity of financial allocation because of established revenue expenditure commitments, makes substantial changes slow and difficult to achieve.

The failure of the tripartite structure to iron out regional inequalities arose partly because the interdependence of hospital and community facilities was not properly understood. The hospital service worked through numbers of hospital beds and supporting services per thousand population. Thus the Porritt report recommended a ratio of eight beds to one thousand population distributed on the basis of 3.4 acute beds, 0.6 maternity beds, 1.6 psychiatric beds, 2.0 geriatric beds and 0.2 beds for other categories, including infectious diseases.[34] But it gradually became evident to the Ministry of Health that it did not really matter how many beds and accompanying hospital services they allocated: if the community health services were poorly staffed or badly equipped to receive patients back from hospital, then the episodes of both acute and chronic illness in the population were not going to decline. Indeed, a pamphlet on the reorganisation issued by the Office of Health Economics stated that, '. . . the regions themselves have little epidemiological significance',[35] implying that although the NHS is about the provision of health care, the reorganisation had very slender demonstrable links with this duty – it had more to do with administrative convenience. The DHSS would not have shared this view and would have maintained that through the Area Health Authorities and the rest of the new management structure, improvements in both health care and the future planning of the NHS resources would be more effectively managed, because the interests of administration and health care coincided. An examination of the structure and functions of the Area Health Authorities will show the basis for these expectations.

The Area Health Authorities

Ninety Area Health Authorities were set up in England and their boundaries in most cases were identical with those of the metropolitan districts and non-metropolitan counties established by the Local

Government Act 1972, which came into effect on the same day as the reorganised health service on 1 April 1974. The populations served by AHAs ranged from ¼ million to over 1 million. Nineteen Areas with teaching hospitals were designated AHA(T). The Grey Book had identified a preferred size of community for which the full range of personal health and social services could be provided at about ¼ million. There were as a result 34 single-district Areas, 23 Areas divided into two Districts, 16 into three Districts, 11 into four Districts, 3 into five Districts and 6 into six Districts.

The chairman of each AHA was appointed by the Secretary of State and paid a part-time salary. This was a new departure looked on with apprehension by some administrators who felt it would encourage chairmen to take an executive role. In the event it did not seem to have a significant effect on how chairmen saw their role, which, in any case, varied from person to person. Membership of the AHA included local authority, university and professional nominees. Local authority membership was increased to one-third by the Secretary of State, Barbara Castle, in 1975. As far as possible, members were nominated not as representatives for any particular group, but as generalists so that they could make decisions on behalf of the community at large. This attempt to remove partisanship from authorities was not entirely successful, given the strong views held by local authority nominees who were almost invariably county or district councillors, and the likely professional views of the two doctors and one nurse also appointed to AHAs.

A distinctive feature of AHAs' duties was their dual responsibility for planning and providing services. They not only provided comprehensive health services including hospitals, community and domiciliary care, but also studied the health needs of the area, and found out where provision fell below required standards. Each AHA determined policies for provision and found the best way of putting them into effect with the resources allocated to it by the RHA. In addition the AHA gave special attention to planning and providing services in conjunction with the matching local authority(ies). Again, as was the case with the RHAs, there had to be a division of labour because members served on a voluntary basis, giving perhaps two or three days a month to the policy-making and resource allocation matters. The day-to-day executive responsibilities were delegated to the Area Team of Officers (ATO), to individual officers at area level, to the District Management Teams (DMTs) and individual District Officers. The activities handled in the Districts (in other than single-district areas) were the basic services associated with the district hospital, the community health services formerly run by the local authority health departments, and the school health service. These functions will be discussed in Chapter 7. The Area Team of Officers had to coordinate the work of the DMTs, but it also had to advise the AHA on developing area-wide policies, informing them of particular local needs and circumstances to be taken into consideration.

The ATO was composed of the Area Medical Officer, Area Nursing Officer, Area Treasurer and Area Administrator. Each officer had a departmental organisation to support him in carrying out his particular professional responsibilities as well as his duties as a member of the ATO. The Area Medical Officer advised the ATO on health care policies and recommended planning guidelines for the Districts in line with these policies. He also advised the AHA on the interpretation and use of advice from his professional colleagues and promoted research and trials into improving health care methods. He had particular responsibilities for child health services in connection with the local authority, and for developing the work of clinicians in the public health field. The Area Nursing Officer contributed to the ATO on matters of planning and policy, and was particularly responsible for the development of integrated nursing services between the hospitals and the community. She advised on the running of the school nursing services and on staffing provision for residential care institutions in the area. Professional training facilities were also her concern and she advised on nursing personnel policies. The Area Treasurer provided financial advice to the AHA in respect of its budget and expenditure. He prepared the Area accounts and ensured proper adherence to its policies by the Districts, and was responsible for the complete paymaster function, including salaries and wages and the payment of all accounts. The Family Practitioner Committee received financial services from his department. The Area Administrator had several roles. He acted as secretary to the Area Health Authority and coordinator of the Area Team of Officers. He prepared advice for the AHA on the development of area-wide policies, issued policy guidelines to the District Management Teams and implemented approved Area plans. He contributed to the Area Team of Officers on planning and policy and was responsible for coordinating and preparing the AHA's formal planning proposals. He was directly responsible for a number of functions managed by other officers, namely, personnel, supplies, ambulance and capital planning. The Family Practitioner Services Administrator was also responsible to him for some aspects of his job. In addition the Area

Administrator coordinated the work of the Area Works Officer and Area Pharmaceutical Officer. He provided administrative support for all the AHA headquarters activities.

It is clear that if AHAs were to function as an effective link in the chain of delegated authority, much depended on the ATO's ability to moderate policies handed down from the Region in a manner that was sensitive to District circumstances, and that was respectful of the DMTs' sphere of authority. The DMT and ATO officers were on the same managerial level, so the ATO could not give orders to the DMT nor be held accountable for their work. It was (in all but single-district Areas) the DMT and not the ATO which was responsible for the actual operation of health care services. The role of the ATO in relation to the Districts was a monitoring one, which meant that the Area Officers could persuade their counterparts in the Districts to conform to policies, and could interpret AHA intentions to them. But if they were not satisfied with the outcome they had to refer the issue to the AHA for a decision about what action might be taken. In the case of the relationship between the ATO and the Regional Team of Officers, each set of officers was accountable to its own authority, so in no sense did a manager–subordinate relationship exist between them. Regional Officers could give advice and guidance to their counterparts on the ATO and persuade them to act in particular ways, but if they were dissatisfied with the Area Officers' performance, their recourse was only to the RHA, which had to decide what to do.

In AHAs with relatively small populations there were no subdivisions into Districts, and these Areas therefore had no DMTs, District Officers or District budgets. The four members of the ATO were joined by a representative consultant and a representative general practitioner to form an Area Management Team who, in addition to the activities described, also took on the work of a District Management Team (to be described in Chapter 4). This arrangement applied to thirty-four of the ninety AHAs in England and three of the eight AHAs in Wales, i.e. 37 per cent of all AHAs.

The Royal Commission on the NHS

The 1974 reorganisation took nearly two years to be implemented and senior staff either retired early or found themselves in new posts. There was a disinclination by some staff to make the new system work. The years 1975 and 1976 were notable for industrial disputes amongst hospital medical staff, first the consultants followed by the junior staff. 1976 also saw Mrs Castle's attempts to restrict private practice facilities, which will be described in Chapter 8.

In May 1976 Barbara Castle asked Sir Alec Merrison, Vice Chancellor of Bristol University, to chair a Royal Commission on the NHS with the following terms of reference: 'To consider in the interests both of the patients and of those who work in the National Health Service, the best use and management of the financial and manpower resources of the National Health Service.'[36] Such a wide-ranging brief provided the opportunity for the first comprehensive review of the NHS since the Guillebaud Report of 1956. The 16 members of the Royal Commission were drawn from a wide variety of interests. They took three years to deliberate at a cost of £918,000. Evidence was sought from a variety of sources, including six specially commissioned studies. Just as the incoming Labour government of 1974 inherited a reorganisation not of its own making, the new Conservative government elected in May 1979 was obliged to deal with a Royal Commission not of its creation. The main conclusion of the Royal Commission when it reported in July 1979 was that 'we need not be ashamed of our health service and that there are many aspects of it which we can be justly proud'.[37] Nevertheless the Royal Commission was critical of certain aspects of the management of the NHS, saying that there were too many tiers, too many administrators of all disciplines, a failure to make swift decisions and a consequent waste of money. In the light of the government's reaction, which was surprisingly prompt, it is worth stressing that the Royal Commission had made recommendations on a wide range of matters, but it was the management of the NHS which emerged as the crucial issue.

The government's views were contained in a publication entitled *Patients First*[38] published in December 1979. This document, somewhat slender in contrast to the volumes published by the Royal Commission, was devoted to the subject of structural change. The government was concerned that over the five years since 1974 the new organisation had not provided the 'best framework for the effective delivery of care to patients'.[39]

Patients First, a consultative paper, suggested that there should be greater delegation so that decisions were made nearer the patients, that District Health Authorities (DHAs) should be set up, thus removing the Area tier; that the professional consultative machinery should be simplified; that functional management should make way for unit management based on hospitals; and that the planning system should be streamlined. Discussion on whether Community Health Councils should continue was invited. *Patients First* did not offer a blueprint for the future and was nervous of wholesale upheaval, in the light of the considerable cost of the 1974 reorganisation — said to be in excess of £9 million. Regions would be responsible for making the arrangements, but were to stand back as far as possible to allow the new DHAs to thrive.

Districts were to be drawn up according to certain criteria. First, social geography, a concept based on the idea of a natural community supported by well established centres of population and linked transport patterns. Interestingly, local government boundaries, even after the 1974 reorganisation, had not always been sensitive to these considerations. The significance of the district general hospital (DGH) and its catchment area was re-established as a reasonable basis for organising health care. Self sufficiency of services was another reason, leaving conterminosity with local authorities a desirable, but not a necessary criterion. This marked a significant turning away from one of the guiding principles of the 1974 reorganisation.

Patients First set a limit of four months for consultation and the government's intentions were duly published in July 1980 in the circular HC(80)8 *Health Services Development: Structure and Management*.[40] This circular largely endorsed the proposals of *Patients First*, but following the widespread and somewhat unexpected support for CHCs, confirmed their continuing existence for the time being. The holding of consultant contracts at District level recommended by *Patients First* had been challenged and was left unresolved.

The 1982 Reorganisation

The timetable allowed for the second reorganisation was two years, and in due course 1 April 1982 was confirmed as the change-over day, with a completion of the total exercise by the end of 1983. This was achieved. But why had this second upheaval been necessary?

Major new legislation always needs a running-in period, but the 1974 reorganisation was remarkable in that even before the end of that period there was widespread dissatisfaction with the new arrangements. By 1976 the Secretary of State acknowledged the state of affairs in setting up the Royal Commission. That such a costly and large-scale reorganisation of a public service could so quickly seem to be unsatisfactory to most people was notable, even in the accelerating rate of legislative change typical of the last 20 years.

Some of the reasons for failure could be said to be practical, but others were a result of faulty concepts. The theme of the 1974 re-organisation was planning. It had been seen as necessary because of the inability of the tripartite service to meet the needs of the community. Planning would be facilitated by an integrated NHS conterminous with local authorities. Areas were set up with the explicit responsibility of providing strategic plans for their Districts, who in turn were to be more concerned with the day-to-day running of the service. But this scheme of things was unrealistic. As Chapter 4 will show, Districts were, in practice, just as likely to have the ideas about future demands as Areas, particularly since they were stimulated by the frustrations of day to day activity. The difference over planning between Areas and Districts developed into the difference between theoretical assumptions of need based on an analysis of statistics together with the views of professional advisers on the one hand, and practical proposals for improvements based on daily experience on the other.

This difference of viewpoint was exacerbated by the conterminosity issue. On the face of it having common boundaries with county councils (or in metropolitan counties, with district councils) would seem to be sensible. But many of these boundaries were arbitrary and did not reflect the organisation of medical care which in many cases had been in existence for nearly half a century. The traditional DGH catchment area often ignored local authority boundaries. AHA members found it difficult to think strategically and by degrees became more and more detached from the everyday working of the NHS. This they found unsatisfying, particularly when they observed District Management Teams getting on with the management of the service without much reference to them.

If the concepts underpinning planning were found to be suspect, the relationships between managers were on the whole worse. The Area Health Authority was served by two sets of chief officers, the Area Team of Officers (ATO) and the District Management Team (DMT). The DMT were not managerially accountable to the ATO but could be monitored by them. This was resented. Some attempts were made to sort out the roles more satisfactorily, but it was clear that the relationship would always be prone to strain, not least because the ATO had easier access to the AHA and particularly the chairman. But even within Districts reorganisation had caused problems. During the late 1960s considerable efforts were made by personnel officers and support service managers — catering and domestic in particular — to develop their roles. The 1974 reorganisation encouraged this process and District appointments on relatively high grades began to appear everywhere. Given the practical nature of some of these services, local hospital support service managers felt somewhat over-supervised. Furthermore, they were often directly accountable to a District Officer making control by the local hospital administrator more difficult.

The new structure could not operate without a considerable increase in staff, particularly administrative and clerical. The government admitted in 1977 that 16,700 extra staff had been recruited because of reorganisation. All these factors contributed to a climate which welcomed the Royal Commission and *Patients First* with open arms. Even Area members and officers supported their own demise.

The failure of the 1974 reorganisation has often been blamed on the management consultants, McKinseys, and on the Health Services Organisation Research Unit at Brunel University, who had both contributed significantly to the pre-1974 discussions. To be fair, the final arrangements contained in the Grey Book represented something of a compromise of their ideas. For instance, McKinseys did not support the duplication of functions at every level of management and yet professional pressure brought that about. The Brunel Unit had always campaigned for clarity of role relationships and the ambiguities of the District/Area relationships could scarcely be said to be their fault.

Changes since 1982

In 1974 reorganisation was conducted according to nationally agreed rules whereas in 1982 each Region was left to sort out its own arrangements. Although minimum upheaval had been advocated by *Patients First* and subsequently by the Secretary of State, this was scarcely the case in most Regions where many Area and District chief officers lost their jobs only to be reappointed in neighbouring Districts. As in 1974, the cost in human terms and hard cash was considerable.

The first two years of the 1982 reorganisation were beset by doctrinal discussions, particularly around the issue of privatisation. The government, faced with an ever-escalating bill for the health services, was seeking ways of off-loading some of the costs. Proposals included encouraging patients to use private hospitals and nursing homes with consequent incentives for more of such establishments to be set up. There was also pressure for health authorities to contract-out support services such as domestic, laundry and catering to private firms.[41] Financial and manpower cuts in 1983 caused considerable unrest. The government for its part was critical of the quality of management in the NHS. There had been a general impatience with consensus management (managing by mutual consent) which had been seen by many, particularly doctors, as an excuse to procrastinate. Given that no one member of a District Management Team was clearly identified as having responsibility for taking action, the accusation carried some weight. Accordingly, the Secretary of State set up a team, led by Mr Roy Griffiths, Managing Director of Sainsbury's, to advise him privately. They prepared a report over a period of six months which was published in October 1983[42] as the *NHS Management Inquiry*. Griffiths identified a lack of drive in the NHS and he and his team said this was because at each level of management no one person was accountable for action. Consensus management had led to delays in decision making and a lowest common denominator effect by which compromise allowed difficult decisions to be avoided. Professional and functional managers had been given too much scope. Griffiths' advice was to appoint a General Manager at Unit, District and Regional level, possibly for a fixed tenure, who would be responsible for improving the efficiency of the organisation. At DHSS and government level the Griffiths proposals were even more radical, suggesting that the Secretary of State should set up a Health Service Supervisory Board with a Management Board accountable to it. The Supervisory Board would be responsible for determining the objectives and direction of the health service, for approving the overall budget and resource allocation, for making strategic decisions, and for monitoring performance. The Secretary of State would chair the board and other members would include the Minister of State (Health), the Permanent Secretary, the Chief Medical Officer and the Chairman of the Management Board. The Management Board would be the executive arm of the Supervisory Board having particular responsibility for implementation of policies, for giving leadership to management in the NHS, for controlling performance and for achieving consistency and drive over the long term. The Chairman of the Management Board would be vested with executive authority derived from the Secretary of State. He would also be responsible for consultation particularly with Regional chairmen. Griffiths proposed that the Chairman of the Management Board should come from outside the NHS and the civil service.

A month after the publication of Griffiths' proposals, the Secretary of State wrote to chairmen of health authorities asking for reactions to the proposals by 9 January 1984. He confirmed his determination to appoint General Managers. In June of the same year Circular HC(84)-13[43] was issued confirming the implementation of the Griffiths proposals forthwith.

The Griffiths proposals stimulated considerable debate, particularly because they appeared to question traditional responsibilities of health authority members and staff. It was not clear whether the Secretary of State saw the proposals as heralding major changes in organisational relationships within health authorities or whether he simply wanted the NHS to work in more action-centred ways. Furthermore, implementation of Griffiths' proposals for the DHSS could be seen to pave the way for fundamental changes in the headquarters' working arrangements.

At the time of writing it was too early to assess the impact of the Griffiths proposals. The DHSS and NHS needed time to consider the observations on such key underlying principles of the 1974 reorganisation as consensus management, the development of professional advisory machinery and the extension of the planning process. Although the Secretary of State had claimed the 1982 reorganisation would allow DHAs to manage their affairs with little interference from above,[44] he was anxious to see more decisive action and progress. Griffiths responded to this by proposing clearer definitions of responsibility and clearer lines of accountability within the NHS and the DHSS as well as between the NHS and DHSS. Linking Griffiths' advice to measures for enhancing effective budgetary management gave the Secretary of State the basis for expecting the health service to do a better all-round job and offer better value for money. Whether this was a realistic expectation will be discussed in the final chapter.

Notes

1. Ministry of Health, Consultative Council on Medical and Allied Services. *Interim Report on the Future Provision of Medical and Allied Services* (Chairman, Lord Dawson), HMSO, London, 1920.

2. Ministry of Health. *Hospital Survey*, HMSO, London, 1945 and 146. (Separate reports on the ten areas of England and Wales.)

3. Parliament. *Social Insurance and Allied Services*. Report by Sir William Beveridge. HMSO, London, 1942 (Cmnd. 6404).

4. Ministry of Health and Department of Health for Scotland. *A National Health Service*. HMSO, London, 1944 (Cmnd. 6502).

5. *National Health Service Bill*, HMSO, London, 1946 (Cmnd. 6761).

6. *The National Health Service Act, 1946*, HMSO, London, 1946 (9 and 10 Geo. 6 Chapter 81 Part I Section I. (1).

7. Ministry of Health. *Report of the Committee of Enquiry into the Cost of*

the National Health Service (Chairman, C.W. Guillebaud), HMSO, London, 1956 (Cmnd. 9663).

8. Medical Services Review Committee. *A Review of the Medical Services in Great Britain* (Chairman, Sir A. Porritt), Social Assay, London, 1962.

9. Ministry of Health. Central Health Services Council. Standing Medical Advisory Committee. *The Field Work of the Family Doctor* (Chairman, Dr Annis Gillie), HMSO, London, 1963.

10. Ministry of Health. *Report of the Maternity Services Committee* (Chairman, Earl of Cranbrook), HMSO, London, 1959.

11. Ministry of Health. *A Hospital Plan for England and Wales*, HMSO, London, 1962 (Cmnd. 1604).

12. Department of Health and Social Security and Welsh Office. Central Health Services Council. *The Functions of the District General Hospital*, Report of the Committee (Chairman, Sir Desmond Bonham-Carter), HMSO, London, 1969.

13. Ministry of Health and Scottish Home and Health Department. *Report of the Committee on Senior Nursing Staff Structure* (Chairman, B. Salmon), HMSO, London, 1966.

14. Ministry of Health. *First Report of the Joint Working Party on the Organisation of Medical Work in Hospitals* (Chairman, Sir G. Godber), HMSO, London, 1967.

15. Ministry of Health. *The Administrative Structure of Medical and Related Services in England and Wales*, HMSO, London, 1968.

16. *Report of the Committee on Local Authority and Allied Personal Social Services* (Chairman, F. Seebohm), HMSO, London, 1968 (Cmnd. 3703).

17. *Report of the Royal Commission on Local Government in England, 1966-1969* (Chairman, Lord Redcliffe-Maud), HMSO, London, 1969 (Cmnd. 4040).

18. *Local Government Finance*. Report of the Committee of Enquiry (Chairman F. Layfield Q.C.), HMSO, London, 1976 (Cmnd. 6453).

19. Department of Health and Social Security. *The Future Structure of the National Health Service*, HMSO, London, 1970. In Wales there was a separate publication: Welsh Office. *The Reorganisation of the Health Service in Wales*, HMSO, Cardiff, 1970.

20. *Reform of the Local Government in England*, HMSO, London, 1970 (Cmnd. 4276).

21. Department of Health and Social Security. *National Health Service Reorganisation: Consultative Document*, DHSS, London, 1971. In Wales, there was a separate publication: Welsh Office. *Consultative Document: National Health Service Reorganisation in Wales*. Welsh Office, Cardiff, 1971.

22. *Local Government in England*, Government Proposals for Reorganisation, HMSO, London, 1971 (Cmnd. 4584).

23. The fruits of Brunel University's HSORU's work are contained in two books: *Hospital Organisation*, Heinemann, London, 1973 and *Health Services*, Heinemann, London, 1978.

24. *National Health Service Reorganisation: England*, HMSO, London, 1972 (Cmnd. 5055). In Wales there was a separate publication: *National Health Service Reorganisation in Wales*, HMSO, Cardiff, 1972 (Cmnd. 5057).

25. *The National Health Service Reorganisation Act, 1973*, HMSO, London, 1973 (Eliz. II Chapter 32).

26. Department of Health and Social Security. *Management Arrangements for the Reorganised National Health Service*, HMSO, London, 1972. In Wales there was a separate publication: Welsh Office. *Management Arrangements for the Reorganised National Health Service in Wales*, HMSO, Cardiff, 1972.

27. DHSS Circular HRC(73)3 *Management Arrangements for the Reorganised NHS*, January 1973.

28. Department of Health and Social Security. *Democracy in the National Health Service*, HMSO, London, 1974. In Wales there was a separate paper: Welsh Office. *Making Welsh Health Authorities More Democratic*, HMSO, Cardiff, 1974.

29. Medical Services Review Committee, *A Review of the Medical Services in Great Britain* (Chairman, Sir A. Porritt), Social Assay, London, 1962.

30. Ibid., p. 23, para. 88.

31. For example, through the publication of the 'Grey Book' which became known, in some circles, as 'the bible'.

32. *National Health Service Reorganisation: England*, HMSO, London, 1972 (Cmnd. 5055), p.v.

33. The Report of the Royal Commission on Local Government emphasised that *all* the needs of a locality should be considered when deciding on boundaries. The difficulties that have resulted since 1974, because in reality the boundaries of AHAs and districts were not coterminous with local authority boundaries in several places, cannot be ignored.

34. Op. cit., *A Review of the Medical Services in Great Britain*, p. 99, para. 367.

35. *The NHS Reorganisation*, Office of Health Economics, London, 1974.

36. *Royal Commission on the National Health Service*, HMSO, London, 1979 (Cmnd. 7615).

37. Ibid., p. 27, para. 3.23.

38. Department of Health and Social Security and Welsh Office. *Patients First*, HMSO, London, December 1979.

39. Ibid., para. 1.

40. DHSS Circular HC(80)8. *Health Services Development: Structure and Management*, July 1980.

41. DHSS Circular HC(83)18. *Health Services Management: Competitive Tendering in the Provision of Domestic, Catering and Laundry Services*, September 1983.

42. *The NHS Management Inquiry* under the chairmanship of Mr Roy Griffiths was commissioned by the Secretary of State in February 1983 to give advice 'on the effective use and management of manpower and related resources' by June 1983. Originally no report was intended but this attracted considerable criticism leading to a change of mind by the Secretary of State. On October 6th a report was sent to the Secretary of State in the form of a letter. It was published two weeks later.

43. DHSS Circular HC(84)13. *Health Services Management: Implementation of the NHS Management Inquiry*, June 1984.

44. *Patients First*, p. 2, para. 5.

2 CENTRAL GOVERNMENT AND THE NATIONAL HEALTH SERVICE

The Functions of Government Departments

The DHSS is not the top tier of the NHS. It is part of government and exists to serve the ministers of the day.

Governments need departments which will transform their laws and policies into action, and thus enable the balance of political power to have its influence on the life of ·the country. In Great Britain each government department is headed by a politician who is either called a Minister or a Secretary of State. He is appointed by the Prime Minister who determines how long he holds that office. If the Prime Minister changes or the government is voted out of office, the political heads of departments also change. However, the permanent staff of the department, the civil servants, continue their work irrespective of alterations in political leadership, and usually spend most of their careers within the department. Although the Secretary of State is the statutory head of the department, he will almost invariably be assisted by a number of junior ministers who are Members of Parliament and also appointed by the Prime Minister.

There are substantial differences between civil servants and politicians over what they want the department to achieve, and in particular, over the time-scale for achievement. Ministers will usually want to establish a number of specific changes in the work of the department during their time in office, to follow the policies of their own party and the views of their fellow MPs. On the other hand, civil servants, because of their longer association with the department, are able to envisage longer term programmes for change. Although the civil service is free from overt party-political domination, it would be naive to assume that civil servants do not have value systems which may well be different from those held by ministers. Those important but rather nebulous factors, personality and style, influence the relationship; the result can be anywhere on the spectrum from close and trusting cooperation to icy formality and deadlock. Whatever the result is, it will influence the department's achievements enormously. A key figure in this is the most senior civil servant, the Permanent Secretary who is generally in day-to-day contact with the Secretary of State. He is, on behalf of the Secretary of State, responsible for the overall management and control of all aspects of the department's administration; therefore the Secretary of State needs to consult him in order to remain well-informed about his department's activities.

The Emergence of the DHSS

The DHSS was created in 1968 from the merging of the Ministries of Social Security and Health. (The origins of the Ministry of Social Security go back to 1916 when the Ministry of Pensions was established. A Ministry of National Insurance was created in 1944 and these two were amalgamated in 1954. Then in 1966 they were joined by the National Assistance Board to form the Ministry of Social Security.) When the Ministry of Health was first formed in 1919, it had responsibility for roads, national insurance, planning, environmental health and local government as well as the health services, but over the years these other duties were transferred to other departments. The final change came in 1951, when it lost responsibility for local government housing to the Ministry of Town and Country Planning, which was itself absorbed into the new Ministry of Housing and Local Government in the same year. This change lost the health ministry its cabinet seat; a loss of status which also meant it had to give up its Whitehall offices and half its staff.

In 1968 Richard Crossman, Lord President of the Council and Leader of the House of Commons, was involved with the Prime Minister in planning the restructuring of certain government ministries that would further consolidate the total number of spending departments. The new Department of Health and Social Security was created in this way, with the Cabinet seat restored (although Enoch Powell was, as Minister of Health, a member of the Cabinet in 1962). The first Secretary of State for Social Services, as the head of the new department was called, was Richard Crossman himself. But the merger did little to alter the organisation of the two ministries since their functions and methods of working were and remained so strikingly different. The former Ministry of Health was a headquarters administration for each arm of the tripartite structure, with the detailed fieldwork in the hands of the hospital boards, executive councils and local authorities. After 1974 the health side of the DHSS employed over 5,000 civil servants, although the actual running of the NHS from day to day was delegated to the health authorities and their staff. On the other hand, the social security side had a much smaller headquarters staff (about 2,000 after 1974) but it employed over 75,000 civil servants in the local offices to administer the range of benefits and welfare provisions on its behalf. Since 1979 the number of civil servants on the health side has been reduced from 5,006 to 4,020 and continues to decline. The Secretary of State himself is a Cabinet minister and has other ministers to help him. There is a Minister for Health and a Minister of State for Social Security. In addition, two or three Parliamentary Under Secretaries of State are appointed with particular responsibilities such as the disabled, health exports, personal social services. The civil servants at the DHSS are organised into two distinct groups, those concerned with health and those dealing with social security, but there is a cross-sector policy group to allow discussion between the two sides. The Secretary of State is also responsible for the Supplementary Benefits Commission which is a separate entity whose commissioners are neither civil servants nor MPs.

The Role of the Health Ministers

The Secretary of State's obligation towards the officers of his department and towards his colleagues in the government can often be conflicting. The department will want him to put its case in the Cabinet, where he has to argue for the government's attention and for funds, in order to support departmental needs and priorities. The Prime Minister and the Cabinet, on the other hand, will require the Secretary of State to be a political force, contributing and supporting the government on matters away from his immediate responsibilities, experienced in Parliament and active in the party organisation. So the person who holds the position of Secretary of State has to achieve a balance between these factors which will, ideally, enable him to be successful, both in his department as an innovator and administrator, and in the government as a politician. As government departments have greatly expanded their activities, increasing amounts of policy preparation have to be done by civil servants, and the minister may at best only be able to choose between policies presented to him by the senior officials, without knowing the details of departmental views on the subject.

Although this might be undesirable from the politicians' point of view, it is an inevitable consequence of the sheer quantity of work being handled in the department. For his own part the minister may call in a group of policy advisers from outside the civil service who will, with his junior ministers, form a team as a countervailing influence to the civil servants.

The Reorganisation of the DHSS

In 1970 the government ordered a study of the DHSS to be made which would, in the light of the earlier reorganisation of the Personal Social Services and the imminent reorganisation of the NHS, make recommendations for a reorganisation of the health side of the DHSS itself. This was carried out by a Review Team under the guidance of a steering committee. The team was jointly composed of civil servants and of management consultants from the firm McKinsey & Company Inc., and the steering committee, chaired by the Permanent Secretary, included senior departmental officials, an Under Secretary from the Civil Service Department, a director of McKinsey and three independent advisers. The Review Team's report was published (in eight volumes) in June 1972,[1] fully accepted by the government and the DHSS, and implemented on a single date in December 1972. Clearly the changes could not, in reality, be as sudden as that, but the intention was to lay the foundations, and simultaneously to build up the organisation upon them, so that the DHSS would be well prepared to guide all parts of the NHS through their reorganisation in 1974. The Review Team's report, like much of the other official literature on the NHS reorganisation, uses a particular vocabulary and style which can easily seem ambiguous and confusing. Although the Department undoubtedly appreciates the need to communicate effectively with those working for the health service, it has often appeared unable to make its meaning plain, and this created a lot of uncertainty, especially in the early months of 1974. So although it is important to have some idea of the way the DHSS works in order to understand how its control of the health service is exercised, the official literature does not make this easy.

The health and personal social services side of the DHSS was reorganised into five groups. Regional Liaison, Services Development, Finance, Personnel and Works, plus the 'Top of the Office' which is made up of department heads (see Figure 3). These groups are supported by the DHSS's own professional advisory staff of doctors, nurses, dentists, welfare officers and social workers. An innovation of the 1972 reorganisation within the DHSS was the Regional Liaison

Figure 3 *Organisation of Functions in the DHSS — 1983*

TOP OF THE OFFICE

To help the Secretary of State provide central leadership in the health and social services.
To advise him on ultimate choices about the nature and scale of the NHS and national objectives and priorities.
To advise him on matters of major public concern.
To manage the Department's resources.

FINANCE

To represent the Department with the Treasury and the rest of government on financial matters.
To provide financial advice to the Top of the Office.
To provide financial advice to the Department as a whole and to review the financial implications of proposed and current policies.
To exercise financial control of the income and expenditure of the Department, the NHS and other agencies under DHSS supervision.
To support the Secretary of State in relation to allocated matters.

SERVICE DEVELOPMENT

To help the Secretary of State decide national objectives, priorities and standards for the health and social services, and specifically to
— Advise on nature and scale of the NHS
— Develop policy needed to improve health services
— Promote local authority social services
— Identify and develop plans to meet needs of selected clients.
To support the field authorities and the Regional Division in implementing these decisions.
To support the Secretary of State in relation to allocated subjects.

REGIONAL

To guide the health authorities on national objectives and priorities.
To support and (to the extent feasible and desirable) control them in the planning and running of services.
To provide specialist support to them in building and supply.
To support the Secretary of State in relation to allocated subjects.

WORKS

To set building and engineering standards.
To determine building and engineering cost allowances.
To develop experimental projects.
To advise on works management and staff training.
To advise on estate management.
To set safety standards.

NHS PERSONNEL

To help the Secretary of State decide fair and economic pay and conditions of service for all NHS personnel, and to see agreement is reached with staff concerned.
To help the NHS recruit, train, retrain and employ wisely sufficient staff of the required calibre and experience.
To support the Secretary of State in relation to allocated subjects.

Group which has had an important function in bridging the gap between the NHS itself and the DHSS and government. Recently, much younger and more able civil servants have been assigned to this work.

The Health Services Development Group has eight divisions which look at broad categories of service and also have a responsibility for particular areas such as children, the mentally ill, the disabled. The Group is concerned with the formulation of policy and with how it is implemented.

The Personnel Group has four divisions, three of which are concerned with all aspects of the pay and conditions of NHS staff that are negotiated through the Whitley Council system. The fourth division deals with doctors' pay and conditions, and the administration of the family practitioner services. The Finance Group has one division dealing with negotiations with central government for the Department's share of money through the PESC[2] system, and one division dealing with allocations to the health authorities, accounting systems and the NHS audit. The Works Group has exerted considerable influence, not always with the full support of other civil servants or non-works staff in the NHS.[3] It has a particular responsibility for giving technical advice to the NHS, for encouraging common standards and for stimulating research into new construction and engineering methods. The Top of the Office consists of the most senior civil servants who advise ministers directly on important matters of policy. In addition, each minister and Permanent Secretary has his own private office which acts as the channel of communication with the rest of the Department and also handles correspondence and arranges meetings and visits.

In 1976, three regional health authority chairmen conducted an investigation into the work of the DHSS in relation to the RHAs, at the invitation of the Minister of State for Health, Dr David Owen. They assessed the performance of the five groups and made a number of radical suggestions for 'encouraging delegation, eliminating duplication and effecting economies'. In response, a joint working group was established to recommend to the Secretary of State what action should be taken on the proposals. In January 1977, before the working group had reported, a further investigation into the work of the DHSS was announced. It was not so much concerned with the relationship between the Department and the health authorities as with improvements in the top management of the DHSS. The inquiry was conducted by senior officials from the DHSS and the Civil Service Department with help from outside consultants. Although the 1982 reorganisation put much of this work in abeyance, the Griffiths report eighteen months later revived the discussion. With the introduction of the Health Services Supervisory Board the internal organisation of the DHSS again became a key issue and it seemed likely that the 1972 arrangements would be modified.

The Personal Social Services

The reorganisation of the DHSS also emphasised the relationship between the personal social services and the NHS. Although the metropolitan districts and non-metropolitan counties are locally responsible for the provision of personal social services which are not part of the NHS, they act under the general guidance of the Secretary of State. Within the DHSS there is a small section of staff working in the social work service, and their influence on health service policy is potentially far-reaching. The welfare of children and people suffering from long-term illness and handicap depends on the liaison between health and social service agencies, and departmental responsibility for supporting and encouraging it is vital in the years ahead.

Monitoring DHSS Activity

The DHSS has to make its case to the Treasury for the resources it believes it needs each year. This gives the Treasury the power to question in detail the DHSS's proposals. Hard bargaining typifies these discussions and major disagreements may arise. For its part, Parliament keeps a check on departments too. Their annual accounts are passed to the Comptroller and Auditor-General who is an independent officer of Parliament. He audits the accounts and reports to the House of Commons, drawing attention to any waste or inefficiency that he has detected. These points will be taken up by the fifteen MPs who are members of the Public Accounts Committee. They hear evidence from the Accounting Officer of the Department (who is the Permanent Secretary) and members of his staff, and recommend ways in which they decide the Department could work more economically or administer its affairs more efficiently. The other instrument of control is the Social Services Committee, a Select Committee of the House of Commons made up of MPs from government and opposition parties. It hears evidence from departmental officials and also from those in the field, and provides its critical assessments to the House of Commons. This combination of the Secretary of State's personal responsibility to Parliament, the Treasury's involvement in departmental planning, the investigations of the Comptroller and Auditor-General, the Public Accounts Committee and the Select Committee provides a basis for thorough and ongoing scrutiny of the Department's work. It is interesting to note that this system has been operating effectively in many aspects of government administration without interfering with ministerial responsibility and authority, or making judgements on party lines.

As monitoring of central government grew more vigorous it became essential that a similar process be adopted between the government and the NHS. Following the 1982 reorganisation a system of ministerial reviews was set up. Each Regional Chairman is summoned to meet one of the ministers once a year. Each side is supported by its most senior officers. The reviews aim to check on the overall performance of the RHA in discharging its statutory duties, to note how far the RHA has implemented government policies and to discuss the Region's plans for particular groups of patients such as the elderly or the mentally handicapped. Ministers may wish to know how successful particular DHSS and government initiatives have been. Recent topics have included the scheme to hasten the discharge of all children from mental handicap hospitals, the scheme to encourage partnership with voluntary bodies in the provision of care and the considerable emphasis being given to joint financing schemes aimed at financial cooperation with social services departments. The reviews are not exclusively about patient care. Following the publication of *Underused and Surplus Property in the National Health Service* (Ceri Davies report)[4] in 1983 which suggested that NHS land was being wasted, the Ministers showed considerable interest in health authority schemes for land disposal or re-use.

Ministerial reviews are not necessarily one sided; they also provide Regions with an opportunity to tell the review team about particular problems within the Region and also to test reactions on new initiatives. Although the actual review meeting is short, the work in preparing for it both in the DHSS and at Regional level is considerable and in itself valuable. The process strengthens the accountability of the NHS to the government — a theme strongly brought out in the Griffiths report. To emphasise this further Regions also have a review process and each District has an annual meeting with the Region, usually on a chairman-to-chairman basis supported by DMTs and RTOs. These may or may not be part of the annual planning cycle; this largely depends upon the timing of the ministerial review itself.

Monitoring is also undertaken by other bodies such as the Hospital Advisory Service (HAS) and the Development Team for the Mentally Handicapped. The HAS was created by Richard Crossman in 1969 following the recommendation in a report of the Committee of Inquiry into conditions at Ely Hospital, Cardiff, for the mentally ill and subnormal:[5] It operated through four multi-disciplinary teams: two for mental handicap, one for mental illness and one for hospitals for the elderly and chronic sick. These teams visited hospitals and units all over England and Wales, and inquired into the details of their day-to-day activities. After each visit they would write a report which was sent in confidence to the hospital authorities and senior staff concerned, as well as to the Secretary of State. The authorities would then discuss the report with the DHSS and agree on responsibility for implementing the recommendations. In 1972 one mental handicap team was disbanded and a second team set up for the elderly, but when the NHS reorganisation was imminent, HAS activity was reduced to just two teams – one for the elderly and one for mental illness. In 1976 the HAS was changed into the new Health Advisory Service to work through joint multi-disciplinary teams with the Social Work Service of the DHSS. These five- or six-member teams look at hospital services, community services and the links between the two. There are two teams: one for the mentally ill, and one for the elderly.

Responsibility for visiting mental handicap institutions in England passed to the Development Team for the Mentally Handicapped which was set up in 1975. This team usually visits by invitation, but can be directed to visit by the Secretary of State himself.

Both the HAS and the Development Team for the Mentally Handicapped set out to encourage and disseminate good practice, new ideas and constructive attitudes and relationships, and to act as catalysts to stimulate local solutions to local problems. They are not able to investigate individual complaints or matters of clinical judgement. Before each visit the DHSS and authorities are asked to supply information about the services to be visited. They are invited to submit their comments, as are the CHCs and Family Practitioner Committees. Senior staff of the health and local authorities concerned, joint consultative committees, staff organisations and any other local bodies may also be invited to make comments. The teams try to reach agreement during the visit on each issue they raise with the staff. Their full report goes to the Secretary of State and the authorities involved. Six months later the health and local authorities are asked about matters raised in the report which have not yet been resolved, and follow-up visits may be made.

The Role of Professional Staff

Returning now to the policy-making duties of the DHSS, a particular characteristic to be considered is the involvement of doctors, nurses and members of other health professions, both as civil servants and in the advisory machinery. They provide expert opinion on the many technical issues involved in the Department's work, and there are Chief Officers of Dentistry, Nursing and Pharmacy, as well as the more well-known positions of Chief Medical Officer and Chief Scientist. They enable the DHSS to approach its work in a multi-disciplinary way, and staff from the Permanent Secretary downwards are acutely aware of the need to take the professionals with them on most policy matters of any substance. The Chief Medical Officer (CMO) is in a particularly influential position since he can consult and advise the Secretary of State personally as of right, without the prior intervention of any other officer and he is likely to be in post for far longer than the ministers or the Permanent Secretary. He works in close liaison with the Permanent Secretary (he has the status of second Permanent Secretary) and he and the other chief officers are consulted on issues that have a bearing on their professional practices and attitudes. The CMO independently publishes an annual report (entitled *On the State of the Public Health*) giving an account of the health care activities of the past year, and in which he can also make his personal comments on the policy and administration of the NHS. These comments are likely to be widely reported and respected. The CMO also has duties as Medical Officer of the Home Office and the Department of Education and Science, and he advises on medical matters to the Ministry of Agriculture, Fisheries and Food, and the Department of the Environment. Such pre-eminence being given to one member of a particular profession is unique within the Civil Service, and is a significant acknowledgement of the medical profession's power and influence. Sir George Godber was Chief Medical Officer from 1960 to 1973, and this exceptionally long service, coupled with his personal reputation and dedication, made the post unusually influential on NHS policy.

The tradition of involving professional opinion and advice in the work of the DHSS is also maintained through advisory machinery. The National Health Service Act 1948 established a Central Health Services Council to advise the Minister on any matters relating to the service that were either referred to them or that they themselves thought fit to consider. After the 1974 reorganisation, this Council was retained, but with a modified constitution. It was made up of between 40 and 44 people: the Presidents of the 13 royal medical colleges (e.g. physicians, surgeons, obstetricians and gynaecologists); 23 professional representatives (e.g. family practitioners, nurses, social workers and health administrators); four representatives of the public; up to four more could be appointed by the Secretary of State. They published an annual report to the Secretary of State, describing the issues they had considered, and they published additional reports on particular matters, which often received publicity in the general and specialist press, and were sometimes discussed in Parliament. Five Standing Advisory Committees of the Central Health Services Council (for medical, dental, pharmaceutical, ophthalmic, and nursing and midwifery services) also looked into issues that had particular reference to their professional sphere, and published reports. These bodies together supplemented the knowledge available to the DHSS and were used as a vehicle to obtain wider support for a new departure in policy, or to strengthen the Secretary of State's position in taking decisions on specific controversial matters. For the first twenty-five years of their existence, these bodies rarely deliberated on matters of their own choosing, but many of their published reports are recognised as important contributions to developments in the National Health Service (e.g. the Bradbeer Report,[6] the Platt Report,[7] the Bonham-Carter Report[8]). Following the 1979 Conservative government's decision to scrap many so called quangos (semi-independent bodies set up by government) the CHSC was disbanded by the Health Services Act 1980.

The Relationship between the Government and the NHS

Since 1948 the NHS has become the keystone of the British welfare state and many people feel that it should not therefore be subject to the vagaries of party politics. The NHS is widely regarded as a powerful symbol of post-war British achievement. But this cannot divorce the NHS from the political system which pays for the service. Politics is about making choices and the NHS is completely dependent on these choices. Within the political system there are tensions between the government supported by the civil service, and the NHS. At times the NHS will feel it is being asked to make changes in the short-term interests of a government, but equally a government may feel thwarted by the apparent inertia of an NHS seemingly devoted to the maintenance of the status quo. It may help to examine these dilemmas in more detail by looking at policy making, allocation of resources and accountability.

Policy Making

A simple view of the role of the government and DHSS in relation to the NHS is that they make policy and pass it down for the NHS to implement. To accept this would be to ignore the vital question, where do policies come from?[9] If a new policy represents a change of direction or a change in the way of doing things, it will often have been stimulated by those who are doing the job already. It therefore follows that policies affecting the NHS are likely to have come *from* the NHS *to* the government rather than vice versa. Even expert committees, often a source of policy change, are usually made up of practitioners and service users. If policy comes from below, it will be influenced by what is possible, and what is possible will be determined by what is acceptable. The government, therefore, is not independent of the influence of the NHS in the policy making process, nor is the DHSS, the government's agent, likely to make much progress if it makes the wrong assessment about what the NHS will tolerate.

During the late 1970s the government and the DHSS increasingly seemed to accept these constraints. Whereas in *Priorities for Health and Personal Social Services in England*[10] expressed intentions for care groups in very specific terms, the follow up document *The Way Forward*[11] was somewhat vaguer. By 1981 when *Care in Action*[12] was published there was almost total acknowledgement that it was up to health authorities to sort out their own priorities within a generalised statement of government intent. The overriding concern then became financial and no significant policy initiatives for care groups emerged during the next two years.

Allocating Resources

Cooperation can be bought. The NHS is much more likely to accept change if a new policy is accompanied by the resources to finance the change. Chapter 6 discusses the contribution which joint financing has made in the development of community based services. In 1983 special funds were set aside to encourage the discharge of children from mental handicap hospitals,[13] and for cooperation with voluntary bodies. In these two cases policies were underwritten by cash. However, this process is not always successful. In 1976 the government set aside £2.5 million a year for regional secure units for those patients needing treatment under greater security than normally available in an average psychiatric hospital. Eight years later few such units exist, held up because of professional differences as to suitable patients and because of nursing union opposition.

Furthermore the general trend of the government has been away from special allocations so that this method for achieving change is now very limited. Chapter 6 will show how the development of financial equity through RAWP and the insistence on cash limits has forced authorities to cope within their existing allocations even though, given the overall popularity of the NHS, individual health authorities' power to embarrass the government should not be underestimated.

Accountability

All spending departments are accountable through their Minister to Parliament. Whilst this may be a correct constitutional statement, the reality is rather more complex. It is impractical to expect the Secretary of State to take responsibility for all that happens in the NHS. If this were so, the long-stay hospital scandals of the 1970s, starting with the Ely Hospital affair (1969) would have led to repeated resignations of ministers. Richard Crossman, the Minister at the time, took the view that his job was to set up an enquiry and demonstrate that the necessary corrective action would be taken.[14] In effect he was holding the NHS accountable to him so that in turn he could answer for the NHS in Parliament.

In the discussions before the 1982 reorganisation it was stressed that there would be an increasing amount of local autonomy as far as decision making was concerned. *Patients First* (1979) enshrined the 1974 reorganisation slogan 'maximum delegation downward, maximum accountability upward', and particularly emphasised the delegation downwards. 'We are determined to see that as many decisions as possible are taken at the local level . . . with minimum intereference by any central authority, whether at region or in central government departments'.[15] After the 1983 General Election the emphasis on accountability of the NHS to the Secretary of State was increased. It seemed that ministers preferred a simple chain of command through chairmen of DHAs to chairmen of RHAs to the Secretary of State himself. This was difficult to carry through in practice given that local authority members of DHAs are not appointed by the Regions but by their own authorities and are not therefore subject to the same controls or disciplinary measures potentially available to bring other DHA members to heel. A dispute regarding manpower and other cuts in one District demonstrated that a DHA cannot be held rigidly account-able by the Region or Secretary of State. A previous dispute regarding an overspending London Area Health Authority had also been an embarrassment to the Secretary of State of the day, Patrick Jenkin, when it was found that the hospital commissioners he had sent in to take over the responsibilities of the AHA (who had been sacked by him) were in fact illegally appointed by him.

The desire to simplify the chain of command may have satisfied some people, suspicious of the way the NHS goes about its decision making, but it left unanswered the question: why set up DHAs at all if their only task is to implement policy passed down from above; health service officers could do the job on their own. In reality, DHAs are also there to serve the local community and in doing this they are bound to challenge the relatively remote centralised viewpoint of the Secretary of State or the DHSS civil servants. With considerable justifi-cation, DHAs can claim that their local knowledge makes them the best people to decide on policies and priorities, even if they accept the constraints such as cash limits imposed by central government. This local awareness and bias gives them a special credibility not available to the Secretary of State.

The tension between the centre and periphery therefore remains. The Royal Commission discussed the possibility of organising the NHS differently.[16] In particular, the lack of direct political accountability to the local community has led to recurring suggestions that the NHS should be run by local government. The opposition to this proposal within the NHS has always been considerable and with increasing central government control of local government, it is not now self evident that the NHS would gain more independence if run by local authorities. A more independent corporation was considered by the Royal Commission but rejected because it might tempt the NHS to assume too much autonomy which would make essential government control much more difficult. At an organisational level it seems likely that the present relationship between central government and the NHS, however uneasy, will remain for some considerable time.

Notes

1. DHSS. *The DHSS in Relation to the Health and Personal Social Services.* Review Team Report. Volume 1. HMSO, London, 1972.

2. PESC is the Public Expenditure Survey Committee – the focus of annual negotiations between spending departments and the Treasury. See discussion in Chapter 6.

3. In 1984 a study team examining the works functions (Chaired by Dr N.J.B. Evans, Deputy Secretary at the DHSS) had difficulty in reaching agreement particularly on matters of managerial status of works officers.

4. DHSS. *Underused and Surplus Property in the National Health Service* (Ceri Davis Report). HMSO, London, 1983.

5. DHSS. *Report of the Committee of Inquiry into Allegations of Ill-treatment of Patients and Other Irregularities at the Ely Hospital, Cardiff*, HMSO, London, 1969 (Cmnd. 3975).

6. Ministry of Health. Central Health Services Council. *Report of the Committee on the Internal Administration of Hospitals* (Bradbeer Report), HMSO, London, 1954.

7. Ministry of Health. Central Health Services Council. *The Welfare of Children in Hospital* (Platt Report), HMSO, London, 1959.

8. DHSS and Welsh Office. Central Health Services Council. *The Functions of the District General Hospital* (Bonham-Carter Report), HMSO, London, 1969.

9. Policy making and policy implementation are part of a wider field of policy analysis. Interested readers may find the following books useful: R. Alford, *Health Care Politics*, University of Chicago Press, 1975; S. Barrett & C. Fudge (eds.), *Policy and Action*, Methuen, London, 1981; C. Ham, *Health Policy in Britain*, Macmillan, London, 1982; R. Klein, *The Politics of the National Health Service*, Longman, London, 1983.

10. DHSS. *Priorities for Health and Personal Social Services in England – A Consultative Document*, HMSO, London, 1976.

11. DHSS. *The Way Forward*, HMSO, London, 1977.

12. DHSS. *Care in Action – A Handbook of Policies and Priorities for the Health and Personal Social Services in England*, HMSO, London, 1981.

13. DHSS. Circular C(83)21. *Helping to get Mentally Handicapped Children out of Mental Handicap Hospital*, September, 1983.

14. R. Crossman. *The Diaries of a Cabinet Minister*, Hamilton & Cape, London, 1975. The Diary entry on the Ely report dated 11 March 1969 said 'I was clear in my own mind that I could only publish and survive politically if in the course of my statement I announced necessary changes of policy'.

15. DHSS. *Patients First*, HMSO, London, December 1979, para. 5.

16. *Royal Commission on the National Health Service*, HMSO, London, 1979, pp. 305–307, paras. 19.2b–19.35.

3 THE REGIONS

The Concept of Regional Administration

The next statutory tier of administrative authority in the NHS has been placed at Regional level. In the original pre-1974 arrangements there were Regional Hospital Boards in each of the ten provincial areas whose boundaries had been defined in relation to the universities which had medical schools. London and South East England were covered by the four metropolitan Regional Hospital Boards which together included the twenty-six teaching hospitals situated in London. These Boards represented a definite tier of authority between the Ministry/Department and local managers, but only in relation to the hospital services. Community health and family practitioner services had no regional administration. During the debate on the reorganisation, successive schemes for achieving an integration of the tripartite structure took differing views on the necessity for regional administration.

In the First Green Paper the idea was absent and in the Second Green Paper, the role was limited to planning and advisory functions only. In the Consultative Document however, a strong regional element in the chain of command from the centre to the periphery was proposed. The reason for this trend in thinking was probably caused by the growing conviction of the Ministers and their expert advisers that there was a need for a coordinating body between the DHSS and the Area administration. The reason was that it seemed necessary to reduce the Department's span of control, and to make the NHS less subject to political pressure.

In that sense, the Regional Health Authorities could be said to have succeeded the Regional Hospital Boards by taking over a number of their functions in relation to the hospital sector, including the appointment of specialist medical staff and the distribution of clinical work across the hospitals within the Region, and the planning and management of capital works and expenditure. Although the intention behind the linking of each RHB to a university medical school and teaching hospital was to improve the distribution of medical manpower throughout the country, inequalities between Regions in the standards of provision were strongly evident all the time. The responsibility for failing to iron out these differences seems to be shared by the Ministry/ Department and the RHBs. Not until 1971 did the DHSS begin to allocate revenue funds to the Regions according to a formula that took account of critical local factors such as the projections of population growth. Before then, the statistical information on which comparisons between Regions could be based was not really sufficiently sophisticated to permit meaningful analyses. However, the RHBs did not influence the development and planning of teaching hospital facilities so that there could be greater integration of the hospital service, and the Department did not encourage them to do this.

The relationship between the RHBs and their Hospital Management Committees was also responsible for some difficulties. In Scotland the arrangement was a strict hierarchy of three tiers: Department of Health for Scotland; Regional Hospital Boards; Boards of Management (the equivalent to the HMCs in England and Wales, although they also had responsibility for the teaching hospitals). Each level explicitly gave orders to the subordinate one below it. In England and Wales, although the RHBs received their orders from the Ministry/Department, they were charged with 'general oversight and supervision' of the HMCs in their regions. This led to the paradoxical situation where some HMCs resented the degree of control exerted over them by their RHB, while other RHBs were criticised for leaving their HMCs alone too much, and allowing administration of an inadequate quality to result. The First Green Paper focused on the first of these points when it said '. . . the interest which Regional Hospital Boards have taken in the performance of management functions by Hospital Management Committees, although not outside their statutory powers, may go beyond what was envisaged when the structure was established. Their primary task as originally conceived was planning and coordinating development; their intervention in matters of management has grown out of their responsibility for allocating financial resources, but it is sometimes unwelcome. Confused responsibilities tend to create unsatisfactory relationships.'[1]

On the other hand, following inquiries at Ely and other hospitals which exposed poor standards of care for long-stay patients, RHBs were criticised for being insufficiently involved, and Richard Crossman held them directly responsible for the activities of their HMCs in this respect.

In the White Paper, however, the reasons explicitly given for needing a strong regional tier did not take up these arguments, and discussions on the most desirable extent of control that should be exerted by

Figure 4 *Regional Health Authority Boundaries*

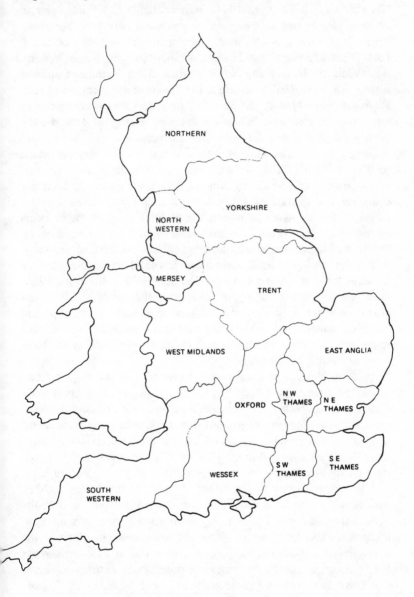

Source: National Health Service Reorganisation, HMSO, 1971

regional authorities over local administration continued vigorously. Nevertheless, from 1 April 1974, fourteen RHAs came into being in England (see Figure 4). The Regions are called Northern, Yorkshire, Trent, East Anglia, North West Thames, North East Thames, South East Thames, South West Thames, Wessex, Oxford, South Western, West Midlands, Mersey and North Western. Their boundaries differed slightly from the RHB boundaries. The chairman and members of each RHA were appointed by the Secretary of State after consultation with interested organisations, including the main health professions, the main local authorities, the universities, appropriate trade unions and voluntary bodies. The work of the RHAs was in some respects similar to that of the old RHBs, including the selection, design and construction of major capital building projects, manpower planning, and major computer and operational research services. But since one important aspect of the 1974 reorganisation was to bring together the elements of the tripartite structure, the RHAs had to look beyond the hospital service to include the community health services in their planning. Although most 'operational' functions were delegated from the Secretary of State through the RHAs to the District Health Authorities, RHAs were responsible for employing consultants and senior registrars, the blood transfusion service, the ambulance service in metropolitan counties, management services, the training of administrators, and for some services better provided on a regional basis (such as the computer processing of payrolls).

In 1979 the Royal Commission suggested that the Regional role should be strengthened even further by making the Regions directly accountable to Parliament. This was rejected in the consultative document *Patients First* on the grounds that it was statutorily inconsistent and would compromise the accountability of the Secretary of State himself to Parliament. *Patients First* went on to reiterate the responsibilities of the Region, but emphasised that they were not to interfere unduly in the day to day affairs of Districts. Monitoring could be used as an excuse to intervene on virtually any matter. Later in the same paragraph comes the first suggestion that a more formal monitoring process should be set up. This was to be developed later in the management advisory service proposals tried out in different ways in four Regions.[2] Another development proposed in *Patients First* was that Districts should have more say in services provided by the Region. It had been usual for Regions to fund services such as computer support, legal advice, public relations, before allocating money to the Districts. Some Regions now first allocate money to Districts and then ask them to agree a level of services to be supplied by the Region. If a District wishes to buy that service elsewhere, for instance legal advice from a local solicitor, they will not pay towards the Regional service. The Region therefore becomes a service-giver and the District, the client.

The members of the RHA are appointed on similar principles to Districts. Before 1974 some Regional Health Boards included HMC chairmen as members. This was believed to tighten up the structure and to a certain extent reduce the differences of opinion between tiers. This arrangement ended after 1974, but *Patients First* suggested that it might be re-examined, and in particular that the majority of members of an RHA should be DHA chairmen. Annual Regional reviews of Districts have been developed since the 1982 reorganisation and are aimed at strengthening the monitoring responsibilities of Regions. The relationship of RHA chairmen to the DHSS will be strengthened by the Griffiths proposals, which say that the chairman of the NHS Management Board 'would ensure that regional chairmen were fully consulted and involved in the discharging of responsibility reserved to the Secretary of State'.[3]

The Regional Team of Officers

The RHA members serve on a voluntary basis and meet about ten times each year, although the RHA Chairman receives a part-time salary in recognition of the extra work which he undertakes. The day-to-day work of the RHA is performed by the five designated officers: the Regional Administrator, the Regional Treasurer, the Regional Works Officer, the Regional Medical Officer and the Regional Nursing Officer. The main work involved is to arrange the distribution of the Region's health service resources in line with nationally and regionally determined policies; in other words, seeing that people, buildings and equipment are in the right place and of the right quality to ensure that the National Health Service can achieve its objectives. For example, this could involve an active policy to reduce the numbers of chronic psychiatric inpatients, or deciding where to site a renal dialysis centre and what its workload should be, or arranging for the right balance between hospital and community care of geriatric patients, and so on. This kind of strategic planning is absolutely necessary in order to spread the limited resources of a Region reasonably across all fronts. The scale of the Regional organisation is large: several of the RHAs

Figure 5 *RHA Work Organisation*

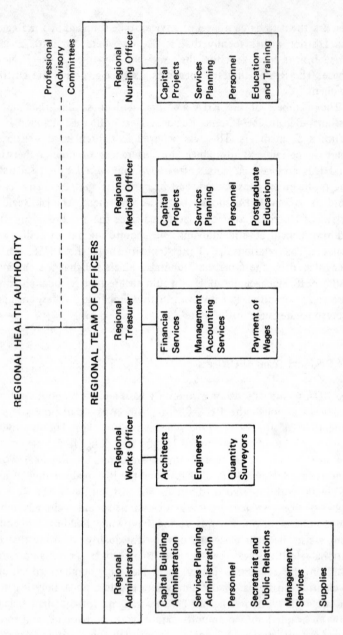

Source: Management Arrangements for the Reorganised National Health Service, HMSO, 1972

serve populations in excess of three million, and in 1983 had annual budgets of between £309m–£848m and staff numbering over 50,000. The management structure focuses on the five designated officers named above. As members of the Regional Team of Officers (RTO) they are collectively responsible for framing regional plans, proposing the allocation of resources, monitoring District Health Authority plans, and providing certain services on a Regional basis. The individual officers have particular specified responsibilities as well, and departmental organisations to support them (see Figure 5).

The Regional Administrator is responsible for preparing plans for the Region's administrative services and seeing that these are carried out. Capital and services planning, personnel, supplies, management services, information services and public relations departments, each with their own senior officer, are managed by him. He also has to provide secretarial services to the RHA, its committees and the Professional Advisory Committee. He manages the services' planning and capital building arrangements and acts as the formal channel of communication between the RHA and the DHSS. The Regional Treasurer is responsible for providing information to the RHA and its senior officers on the capital and revenue implications of the region's work through management accounting and internal auditing systems, and for arranging the computation and payment of wages to staff. He also advises the District Treasurers on the management of their income and expenditure. The Regional Works Officer has a large staff of architects, engineers and quantity surveyors who are involved in the planning of new buildings in the Region, and the maintenance of the Region's capital stock. The Regional Medical Officer is in charge of planning the distribution of medical manpower throughout the Region, and coordinates the work of multi-disciplinary groups which study the development of operational health care services. He has to ensure that medical education and research facilities are suitably developed, through cooperation with the university and teaching hospital authorities, and that personnel services are available for regionally employed medical staff. The Regional Nursing Officer is responsible for the development of nursing standards and ensuring adequate education and training facilities throughout the region. She also contributes, with the other members of the RTO, to the development of plans for health care services and for capital building.

The Regional Team of Officers was a 'consensus-forming' group of equals. The concept of consensus management has been discussed generally, but its definition of the style in which RTOs were meant to work can be seen as an interesting departure from pre-1974 arrangements. The origins of 'consensus' come from academic research into the ways groups of people solve problems together, which has suggested that team methods can often be more effective than either committee or individual efforts, in given situations. Traditionally, the leadership of a committee always rested with the same person, the chairman, who was not necessarily informed about the subjects under discussion. Decisions were taken, when necessary, by majority vote, and this often failed to recognise or reconcile the different opinions of members. The new arrangements, however, required teams to arrive at unanimous decisions after thorough discussion of individual points of view and their respective implications. The consequence was that no one member was necessarily more powerful than another, and that the collective decisions reached were a statement of the members' commitment to the action that resulted from their decision.

Just as the DHSS has arrangements for obtaining expert professional advice, so the RHAs have advisory committees of health service staff which may cover medical, dental, nursing and midwifery, pharmaceutical, optical and other categories of services. These committees enable RHAs to make development plans in consultation with the professions, and ensure the participation of individuals outside the RHA staff in the all important planning process.

Management Relationships and the Planning Process

The architects of the 1974 reorganisation based many of the detailed arrangements for improved administration on the complementary concepts of 'maximum responsibility delegated downwards' matched by 'clear lines of accountability upwards', which would be exercised through the creation of sound management structures at each level. In effect this meant a division of labour between the levels of authority which was designed to ensure that the DHSS' policy intentions would be put into effect, more or less uniformly, across the country. An oversimplified way of saying the same thing is that the DHSS did the strategic planning on a national scale and the RHAs did the strategic planning on a local scale whilst remaining faithful to the DHSS' guidelines. Since 1982 the DHAs handle details of staffing and services that make the RHAs' plans possible, and they deal with the 'delivery' of health care to their populations, with the resources that are made available by the RHAs. The result is that each level allocates resources to the next one down, which in turn redistributes them and passes them on. This delegated responsibility for using resources is mirrored by accountability up through the levels, which is achieved through the medium of plans and budgets. So Districts submit plans to the Regions and Regional plans go to the DHSS. The plans are in each case scrutinised by the 'senior' authority which allocates budgets to cover the items in the plans that have been approved. It thereby sanctions the carrying out of the approved plans by its 'junior' authority. There are paradoxes in this scheme, particularly because the NHS inevitably has to operate in the context of a continuously growing demand for its services. Therefore whatever services are being arranged are likely to fall short of the current level of demand or the state of medical knowledge. This state of affairs forces each level of authority to choose between alternative priorities, since it will never have enough money or staff to provide everything it ideally should. Although national policy envisages a shift of emphasis from the hospital services to the community health services, this cannot easily be achieved with the limitations on available resources, since it would entail allowing the hospital services to deteriorate so that the community services could benefit. Such a move is unacceptable, and the only alternative is to devise ways of using the existing resources more economically thus spreading their effect more widely. 'Sound management structures' are held to be the way that appropriate handling of this delicate situation will be achieved. Nevertheless, there is concern that instead of delegated responsibility being matched by accountability, the pressure on the structure tips the balance in favour of accountability. The effect of this is that higher levels of authority tend to keep too tight a grip on the plans and expenditure of the lower levels so the greater freedom to distribute resources according to local circumstances will be minimised.

In the case of RHAs and their Districts, the Regions have to judge the correct balance between their claims and monitor their subsequent performance according to the approved plans.

There is not meant to be a manager–subordinate relationship between Regional Officers and their counterparts at District level. It is, rather, a matter of the Regional Officer giving advice and guidance on the interpretation of RHA policies in general, and in connection with specific problems which may arise. He is meant to avoid giving the District Officer orders and instead tries to persuade him to get particular things done in particular ways. The relationship between the DHSS and the RHAs is slightly different although adhering to the same general principles. Through its establishment of a Regional Planning

Division the DHSS has attempted to forge much closer and developing links with the RHAs so that it can be in touch with operational problems and trends that will make its picture of the way the NHS works more accurate. There are regular meetings with the RHA chairmen and with particular Regional Officers, and individual RTOs meet with the Regional Planning Division of the DHSS.

Until 1974 there was no formal or explicit planning system in the NHS, and the Department found itself constantly being asked to react to changes and crises that it was not well equipped to understand or deal with. Now its intention is to think ahead and analyse alternative ways of achieving its national objectives, and thereby assign priorities between them for the use of its limited resources. The working of the NHS is in many respects regular and predictable, so a formal planning process is a suitable way to organise its administration. The problem is that there are no objective ways of measuring performance in the service that are equally acceptable, so some of the planning judgements take on the status of informed guesses. Nevertheless, the DHSS operates an annual planning cycle in which each level is simultaneously involved in an ongoing assessment of its targets. The DHSS decides on its priorities with the Secretary of State and then agrees with the RHAs on how these may be broadly achieved. They pass guidelines on to the DHAs that are tailored to fit specific local circumstances, and give an idea of the financial allocations that may be expected. Districts are anyway involved in charting the services that they need to provide for their local populations.

The RHAs' role is to coordinate and approve District plans. Neither the DHSS nor the RHAs should be involved in the detail of District plans, but only in satisfying themselves that the latter fit into the overall strategy at Regional and National levels. Further details of the timing of the planning cycle will follow in Chapter 7.

The Functions of the Region

Planning

The planning function is divided into two main elements, service planning and capital planning. In the early days of the NHS planning was entirely concerned with replacing old buildings with new and *A Hospital Plan for England & Wales* (1962)[4] was almost entirely concerned with numbers of hospital beds. But since 1974 the concern for particular groups needing care has resulted in the development of service planning. Service planning takes a broad view and asks what are the needs of a particular group of the population and in what various ways could these be met? Evaluating alternative options is an important part of the process. A plan for the mentally handicapped, for instance, needs to evaluate the medical, social and resource implications of alternative strategies. Does living in the community provide a higher standard of care, a better quality of life and is it cheaper? All these considerations will be valid for the service planner.

Although it is possible for each DHA to have its own view on these subjects, in order to ensure reasonable equality of service across the country, each DHA's initiative has to be set within the context of an overall national strategy. Regions are the agents through which the DHSS promulgates these strategies. This does not oblige Regional responses to be uniform and particular Regions have developed distinct approaches to particular problems.

Economic theory has progressively influenced service planning through the 1970s and there has been increasing use of the technique of cost-benefit analysis, which attempts to evaluate the social costs as well as the monetary benefits of alternative investments, and the concept of opportunity cost which attempts to evaluate the other opportunities which will be foregone if one particular choice is made. Thus if there is a limited amount of money for developing services for the mentally handicapped, choosing the option of a locally based twenty-five place hostel would preclude spending the money on setting up smaller community homes.

The discipline required for planning in this manner has gone some way to correct the impression that health service developments were controlled by influential power groups. Indeed, developments in the so-called 'Cinderella' services would otherwise have been even more modest, given the demands of the district general hospitals.

The techniques used in service planning arose from a more orderly approach to capital planning which evolved towards the end of the 1960s. The DHSS had been issuing throughout the 1960s a series of *Hospital Building Notes*[5] which laid down design standards for various departments. These were supplemented in 1969 by the *Health Building Procedure Notes*[6] otherwise known as Capricode. Capricode, which every Region has to employ in developing its capital plans, is a step-by-step procedure starting with a case of need and proceeding via various stages such as tender approval and culminating in evaluation. It prevents time and money being wasted through agreeing a contract for a new building and then subsequently altering the plans. Regions organise their planning and development departments to enable

Capricode to operate and project teams consisting of an administrator as coordinator, an architect, a nurse and a doctor, with possibly other works professionals such as an engineer and a quantity surveyor, are allocated responsibility for a geographical part of that Region. The project team works with a similar group of people at District level on all major projects. Smaller capital projects are delegated direct to Districts.

Some Regions have developed their own design expertise and have produced purpose-designed buildings which are marketable beyond their own boundaries. Others have made significant contributions to standard designs such as Nucleus and Harness produced by the DHSS.[7] Not all design work is done in-house, however, and most of the major new hospitals built in recent years have employed architects of national and in some case international repute, some of whom have specialised in this sort of work. In these cases the Regional architect has been responsible for supervising the scheme.

Regional planning and works departments are also responsible for estate management. The Woodbine Parish report of 1970[8] was critical of the poor standard of hospital maintenance and the lack of any overall strategy for the development of health service estates. As a result in 1972 the DHSS produced the first draft of its *Estate Management Practices Code*[9] (Estmancode) which aimed to advise the NHS on the proper procedures for planning and costing maintenance work, for executing maintenance to a proper standard, for ensuring efficiency of plant by improving works department organisation and information and finally for keeping a proper register of land. This last requirement has been of particular interest to recent governments and in 1977 the DHSS issued a *Handbook on Land Transactions*.[10] In 1983 renewed pressure was put on health authorities to capitalise on land holdings, selling off those which were not needed for health service use. At present health authorities are not able to seek redesignation of land, say from agricultural to housing use, and therefore cannot maximise the value of their holdings. Legislation is being passed (1984) to alter this.

Regional engineering departments have been particularly concerned with energy conservation and many Regions have set aside money for this particular purpose.

Resource Allocation

The details of how the funds are allocated by Regions will be found in Chapter 6. Simply, the Regions are required to dispense the money they receive from the DHSS and to do so in a fair manner. The Resource Allocation Working Party (RAWP) was set up in 1975 to review the method of distributing funds and a year later published its report[11] which recommended more flexibility between capital and revenue, a review of data collection methods and further research into the validity of criteria used for evaluating need. This last point was particularly important as RAWP had suggested that an attempt must be made to reach a fairer distribution of funds between Regions, and, it must be supposed, within Regions. Target revenue allocations were recommended taking into account a range of variable factors such as the age, sex, fertility and mortality rates of the population of a Region. The RAWP formula, now used by the DHSS, is not necessarily employed by Regions in allocating funds to Districts, and in any case an unduly rigid view of equity can hinder measures to reduce inequalities. There is no clear relation between the allocation of funds and the quality of service.

One Region with a lower allocation may have lower mortality rates than another. Similar differences can be observed between Districts. Another disadvantage of a rigid adherence to a formula is when a Region has to judge between the needs of particular Districts. For instance, one District may be providing a mental illness service for another. The opening of a major new hospital may require additional funds at least initially, so that a policy of flexible funding is required, allowing variations of allocation over a period of years. Finally, a Region may wish to develop a particular service, and will reserve funds for this purpose because unfunded priorities are less likely to be honoured by Districts.

Monitoring

It has already been said that Regions are expected by the DHSS to ensure that national policies are being implemented using plans and budgets to match downward delegated authority to upward accountability. Until the 1982 reorganisation there was considerable evidence that each District chose its own set of priorities, largely ignoring guidance from above if found unwelcome. Only special earmarked allocations of money could overcome this tendency to a limited extent. Since 1982, the yearly ministerial review has tightened up the monitoring process. Each year the Minister of State (Health), accompanied by some of the most senior DHSS officials, visits each Region, to review progress. Although the visit is short the considerable preparation leading up to it acts as a useful stimulus to the monitoring process. Similarly, Regions conduct a review with each of the Districts. Some Regions can link this with the annual planning cycle which is sensible, but the timing of the Minister's visits to other Regions makes this difficult.

Manpower Control

The Regions are involved with detailed control of two groups of staff. First, administrative staff are controlled through the management cost exercise set up by the DHSS to reduce the overall cost of management within the NHS.[12] By 1983, the government were claiming success in that the amount spent on management had declined from 5.1 per cent in 1979/80 to 4.4 per cent in 1982/83.[13] The Region's second direct manpower concern is with medical staff. Additional medical staff can only be employed if three conditions are satisfied: first, finance, which the Districts must find for themselves; second, manpower approval; third, in the case of posts below consultant, training recognition. The Regions are involved in the last two. Following various attempts to regulate the number of doctors (for details see Chapter 8) the DHSS will only approve certain additional posts in certain specialties and require the Region to administer this process. The Region may think it right to reallocate within the District, so that a consultant or registrar post foregone in one District can be transferred to another. Training standards are set by the medical profession itself and with the introduction of compulsory vocational training for general practitioners, there are now no medical posts exempt from training recognition, except clinical assistants. It is up to Regions to monitor this situation. Districts only have freedom in the appointment of clinical assistants who are employed on a sessional basis to help consultants. They are usually general practitioners wishing to keep some links with hospital medicine.

Other Functions

The functions described above are obligatory for all Regions, but there are others which they can organise to suit themselves, either by delegating to Districts or by developing a central Regional department. These include supplies, management services, training, personnel, legal services, public relations and research.

The supplies function has been much reorganised and will be discussed in more detail in the next chapter. The setting up of the Supply Council in 1980[14] has resulted in instructions to Regions as to how to organise supplies in the future. Some Regions have put the whole supplies function under the responsibility of the regional supplies officer, but others have delegated it to some Districts to manage on behalf of others in the same Region.

Management services includes the traditional work study role as well as the development of computer and information technology. Regions set up computer facilities in the late 1960s mainly to process salaries and wages and keep account of stores. Further applications of computers to medical records then developed, principally through the introduction of Hospital Activity Analysis (HAA) which summarises the basic information held in medical records regarding patient admission, treatment and discharge. Regions now have difficult decisions to make about their objectives for data collection and processing. They need to make plans which link sensibly to District resources; and they need to specify a clear information strategy, not least because of the recommendations of the Körner Committee on health service information.[15]

Training NHS staff to adapt to the constant changes in knowledge and practice is an important responsibility. Some Regions have developed sizeable training departments and give particular emphasis to management training. Some regional training officers run courses with their own staff or use the various training institutions which provide a network across the country, and local colleges and polytechnics are also used. Each year the National Management Training Scheme recruits around 45 young people, many of whom are graduates, for a two-year scheme which is administered by the Regions. Attachments to Districts and to the Regions ensue and the trainees have a thorough grounding in all aspects of NHS management and during their second year have an opportunity to work in a supervised post. Similar schemes operate for finance and supplies trainees in several Regions.

The regional personnel officer is likely to be in overall charge of the development of staff and the training department will be part of his concern. He or she is also concerned with manpower planning and with industrial relations. Staff policies are either determined nationally or they are negotiated in each District. However, trade unions see an advantage in endeavouring to get Regional commitment to certain policies such as time off for trade union activities or the introduction of bonus schemes, because this will be more likely to ensure commitment from the Districts.

Most Regions provide a specialist legal advisory service. The law relating to health matters is a specialised area[16] and it is therefore usual to have a small department in each Region from which Districts may obtain advice. Although the level of litigation in the NHS is low, all health authorities are involved with some and the Regional legal adviser normally acts on behalf of the health authority, often in conjunction with the professional defence society such as the doctors' Medical Defence Union. Legal advisors also give advice on employment law and conduct land and property transactions for the Districts.

The NHS, as a public service authority, is constantly liable to be exposed to public scrutiny. There are many times when this results in 'bad' publicity arising from something which has gone wrong. Traditionally, health administrators have not been particularly skilled in handling the presentation of the NHS to the public and most Regions now have a specialist public relations department.[17] Apart from handling press inquiries the public relations department may try to promote 'good news' stories and to develop a feeling of Regional identity amongst the staff with the publication of an in-house newspaper.

Although much medical research is undertaken in the NHS it is usually funded by voluntary bodies or by drug companies. The DHSS research funds are relatively small so Regions may want to fund projects either undertaken at Regional level or in a local university or a District. For instance, several Regions have undertaken research to support health promotion schemes aimed at reducing the level of smoking, extending the wearing of seat belts and other campaigns. Other research projects have included evaluation exercises of models of care for the mentally handicapped and ward design.

Notes

1. *National Health Service Reorganisation: England*, HMSO, London, 1972 (Cmnd 5055).

2. The management advisory service evolved by the *Reply by the Government to the Third Report from the Social Service Committee. Session 1979-1980*, HMSO, London, 1980 (Cmnd 8086). Three trials were set up in 1982 in the North Western Region, a joint trial between Oxford and the South Western Region, and in the Wessex Region. The format was different in each.

3. *The NHS Management Enquiry*, p. 4, para. 3.

4. Ministry of Health. *A Hospital Plan for England and Wales*, HMSO, London, January 1962.

5. Ministry of Health/DHSS. *Hospital Building Notes*, HMSO, London, 1962 onwards.

6. DHSS. *Capricode – Health Building Procedure Notes*, HMSO, London, 1969.

7. The Nucleus hospital concept was introduced in 1976 to avoid the necessity of building very large district general hospitals in one stage. Under this system a core of beds and services could be added to as capital and extra revenue monies became available: each unit could be 'harnessed' to the next. This method overcame costly monoliths such as the ill-fated Royal Liverpool Hospital, the cost of which, at over £50 million, grossly exceeded the original estimate.

8. DHSS, SHHD, Welsh Office. *Hospital Building Maintenance* (Woodbine Parish Report), HMSO, London, 1970.

9. DHSS. *Estmancode – Estate Management Practices Code for the NHS*, HMSO, London, 1972.

10. DHSS. *NHS Handbook on Land Transactions*, HMSO, London, 1977.

11. DHSS. *Sharing Resources for Health in England* (RAWP Report), HMSO, London, 1976.

12. In 1976 the DHSS imposed limits to reduce the number of administrative staff.

13. House of Commons. Parliamentary Debates, Official Report. *Hansard*, 1 November 1983, p. 366.

14. The Secretary of State under Section 11 of the NHS Act 1977 set up the Supply Council as a Special Health Authority. Its intention set out in circular HC(80)1 January 1980, was to secure better value for money in the procurement of supplies and so to free resources for the direct care of patients.

15. DHSS. *Steering Group on Health Services Information*, chaired by Edith Körner, then vice-chairman of the South Western RHA. Miscellaneous reports from 1982 onwards.

16. The standard textbook is *Speller's Law Relating to Hospitals and Kindred Institutions*, Sixth Edition, H.K. Lewis, London, 1978.

17. Administrators are endeavouring to improve. Some Regions run special courses for handling the media and television appearances. See also the IHSA Management Series No. 8: *You May Quote Me*, Mitchell and Taylor, IHSA, London, 1983.

4 THE DISTRICTS

The present arrangement of Districts in the NHS derives from the consultative document *Patients First* and the DHSS circular HC(80)8[1] which set out in July 1980 how the NHS was to be restructured. Since 1 April 1982, as permitted by the Health Services Act 1980 Section 1, the old Area Health Authorities have been disbanded in favour of 192 new District Health Authorities (DHAs). Although these largely have the same boundaries as their predecessor Districts, there are some exceptions. In particular the largest District of all, Leicestershire, was created out of amalgamations to produce a population of 836,000. There are also a few very small Districts of under 100,000 population, but most are around the 250,000–350,000 population size. Twenty-six Districts have medical schools, but the old special suffix (T) has been removed, perhaps bearing in mind that medical schools use many District General Hospitals for practical experience.

The Functions of the New Districts

Each District Health Authority was to be responsible for 'the planning, development, management of health services in its District within national and regional strategic guidelines'.[2] This advice was amplified in a further circular issued in May 1981 HC(81)6.[3] Specifically, DHAs had to make sure they had integrated plans for the provision and development of primary care, general hospital services, maternity and child health services and also for services for the mentally handicapped, the mentally ill and the elderly. They were to appoint their own chief officers forming a District Management Team (DMT).

Although Area Health Authorities had had similar responsibilities, they had found it increasingly difficult to get a feel for the service because of their remoteness from the previous DMTs. Now with a direct relationship it was hoped matters would be better. The Authority would review and on occasions challenge the proposals put forward by DMTs. It could also ask DMTs to prepare options so that members had a choice to make, thus avoiding the frequent criticism that health authorities were merely set up to 'rubber stamp' decisions already made by their officers.

Before describing the work of the DHA members further, it may be useful to discuss who they were and how they got there.

The Chairman and Members

The chairmanship of each DHA is in the gift of the Secretary of State himself. During the last decade, each government has been accused by its opponents of making political appointments. In fact health authorities before and after 1974 have not acted in a particularly party political way. Some inner city authorities are now conducted on lines similar to a local authority, but for the majority of health authorities debate is usually free of explicit party statements, even, surprisingly, in debates on such subjects as private practice which contain a strong ideological element. As with many other public bodies in England, the selection of a candidate for the post of Chairman of a DHA and indeed of an RHA, is done via the 'old boy' network whereby those in influential positions in society suggest a suitable candidate. Recently attempts have been made to attract people with experience of industry rather than those with more traditional links with voluntary bodies. As the chairman is appointed directly by the Secretary of State, it might be assumed that this implies some sort of personal accountability to the Secretary of State. In fact at District level this does not seem to be the case and chairmen have so far had considerable freedom to lead their DHAs in whatever direction seems to be indicated by local needs and demands.

The Chairman is paid about £9,000 per annum (1983) and he or she is expected to devote about two days a week in aggregate to the District. The manner in which chairmen perform their duties varies considerably. Some are to be found in the District most days, acting almost as a chief executive officer, whilst others attend relatively infrequently, happy to let the DMT get on with running the District. The chairman acts as a bridge between the DHA and its officers, particularly the DMT. In some cases the DHA may feel that the Chairman is more like an officer than a member and for the interested and concerned chairman, this affiliation will be difficult to avoid.

The members are selected from nominations received from several sources. Circular HC(80)8[4] specifies that each authority should include one hospital consultant, one general practitioner, one nurse/midwife/health visitor, one nomination from the Region's medical school, one trade union member, four (or more in certain cases) local authority nominees and seven (or more) other generalist members. A hospital consultant is put forward by his colleagues and can be working in the same District (although his contract is held at Region). Similarly the general practitioner is likely to be put forward by the local medical committee or similar representative group of general practitioners. The nurse should not, however, be a member of the staff of that DHA. This has happened previously and introduced an untenable position since the District Nursing Officer was in effect her or his own employer. Each Region has at least one medical school and one nomination is made by that university, but the person need not be a member of the medical school's staff itself.

The Labour government of 1974–1979 had tried to improve staff representation on health authorities through proposals in their paper *Democracy in the NHS*.[5] Not unexpectedly, the Conservatives subsequently wished to reduce any representation that looked like the first step towards workers' control, so HC(81)6 said that the trade union member need not necessarily be from a trade union affiliated to the TUC. The District's own staff or full-time trade union officers were specifically barred.

Local Authority membership is in practice subject to some negotiation with the Regions. Large Districts may well include more than four county and district councils, so that there has to be some agreement as to who may make the nominations. One way around this problem is to increase the number and this has been done. Local authority members are not subject to a four year tenure of office, although RHA appointed DHA members can serve for more than one term of office. This subtle difference in status was not seen as significant until 1983, when certain DHAs were rebelling against the manpower cuts and financial limits imposed by the government through the Regions. A Region can dismiss all the members of a recalcitrant DHA, except for those from local authorities, who continue to be the nominees of their local authorities even if the Region appoints a new DHA.

This constitutional trial of strength may be a diversion and it is more usual for local authority members to be nominated because they already have experience in kindred services such as social services and education. The remainder of the membership, which must bring the authority up to a minimum of sixteen members, are chosen from a variety of sources. One or two Regions even advertise for members. Care is taken when appointing members to ensure that age, sex, geographical location, profession and political affiliation are reasonably balanced. As a result, the authorities may well be more broadly representative of a community than are elected local authorities even though the health authorities have been criticised for being undemocratic. All the health authorities have difficulty in obtaining nominations for members from young, ethnic minority and working class backgrounds.

How Do DHAs Conduct Their Business?

No rules are laid down for the formation of sub-committees, unlike previously when a financial sub-committee had been required by statute. DHAs are free to arrange their affairs as they think fit, but circular HC(81)6[6] says that it is important to guard against three things: first, a disproportionate increase in administrative workload and expense; second, an erosion of members' corporate responsibility by giving too much authority to small groups of members; third, secrecy by not discussing matters in public. DHAs are reminded that they are governed by the Public Bodies (Admission to Meetings) Act 1960, and Appendix 4 of the circular gives fuller details.

No research has yet been completed on the way DHAs conduct their affairs,[7] but it seems likely that most DHAs have monthly or bimonthly meetings and arrange sub-groups of members to examine particular issues. These groups may be standing sub-committees, but are more likely to be more flexible than that, concerning themselves with monitoring certain aspects of the service and with promoting new ideas on the development of care group strategies.

Agency Services

Some DHAs run services on behalf of others; three in particular are worth more detailed discussion. The reasons for their arrangements vary but are related to the previous history of the services in question. The three are: family practitioners services, supplies and ambulances.

Family Practitioner Services

Family practitioner services are the administrative responsibility of the Family Practitioner Committee (FPC). Each FPC is made up of 30 members, eleven appointed from constituent DHAs, four from local authorities, eight by the local medical committee (one of whom must be an ophthalmic practitioner), three by the local dental committee,

two by the local optical committee (one of whom must be an ophthalmic optician and the other a dispensing optician) and two by the local
pharmaceutical committee. The FPC has to make arrangements for the
provision of family practitioner services and to publish lists of all practitioners undertaking work in its area and to pay those practitioners
under contract with the FPC. Complaints by patients arising from services managed by the FPC have to be investigated too (see Chapter 12).

Following the 1974 reorganisation, family practitioner services
became managed by the FPCs which replaced the old Executive Councils. FPCs were set up in each area as semi-autonomous bodies, although
their corresponding Area Health Authority actually provided the
premises and office services as well as employing the FPC staff.[8]
Following the subsequent reorganisation which led to the AHAs being
abolished, a fresh look was taken at the status of the FPCs. The government decided to make them fully independent special health authorities
in their own right. Pending the necessary legislation to achieve this
certain District Health Authorities were given the job of continuing the support previously provided to FPCs by some AHAs. For this
the DHSS separately allocated Exchequer funds to the DHAs concerned.

The relationship between FPCs and AHAs was always rather ambiguous and the decision to make FPCs fully autonomous still does not
clarify two underlying issues: how can family practitioner services be
fully integrated with the rest of the NHS and social services so as to
provide the best care for patients; and what method of paying the
practitioners and financing their work is most cost-effective? Both
points are crucial to good planning and provision of care.

Supplies

Despite the fact that running the supplies service was one of the main
tasks of a municipal hospital administrator prior to 1948, this function
has never been a popular area (except amongst specialist supplies
officers themselves). This may explain why it has been subject to more
change than most parts of the service. In the 1950s, worries over the
methods and financing of supplies led to the Messer Report 1958[9]
and later to the Hunt Report 1966.[10] Following that, Area Supplies
Departments were set up which served several hospital management
committees to provide an organisation big enough to justify joint
contracting and joint purchasing. Before long, however, the 1974

reorganisation put supplies back within the boundary of each area health authority.

The Three Chairmens' report on the DHSS (1976)[11] was critical of aspects of supplies organisation nationally and the Collier Report[12] in the same year made another attempt to make sense of purchasing arrangements. A further working group, set up under Sir Brian Salmon,[13] produced a report in 1978 which recommended much tighter management of supplies services with all supplies staff being accountable to the Area Supplies Officer, even if they were based in Districts. It recommended setting up a National Supply Council as a special health authority to advise the Secretary of State on supplies matters and, if necessary, impose mandatory decisions on the service. The Supply Council was duly set up in 1982. Then the 1982 proposals for reorganisation put one district in charge of the old Area Supplies organisation on behalf of others. By 1984 this shift in responsibility had largely been achieved, with divisional supplies departments usually serving more than one District and with a divisional supplies officer accountable to the regional supplies officer or in some Regions this was delegated to a managing District. Large central stores are being set up supported by computerised systems. The two different ways of managing supplies, direct by Region or through a managing DHA, will be reviewed and a final decision made in favour of one or the other.

Ambulances and Other Patient Transport

Before 1974 the ambulance service was run by 142 local health authorities (not every health authority ran its own). In 1974 the service was transferred to the new AHAs with the exception of London where the South West Thames Region ran the service for the whole of London and the other six metropolitan counties where the service was run by the appropriate RHA. During the 1970s, the demand for ambulance transport grew, partly because of the growing number of in- and outpatients and partly because public transport, particularly in rural areas, was getting worse. A key question is whether to separate the emergency services, only 5 per cent of all journeys, from the rest and link them to the other emergency services — the fire brigade and the police. In 1980 the DHSS set up a working party on patient transport services under the chairmanship of the outgoing administrator of the Trent Region, Maurice Naylor. The report rejected the idea of a two-tiered service with the possible exception of metropolitan areas, but suggested more could be done to create community transport services for those in need, and this might be a suitable project for collaboration with local authorities. The report was critical of the lack of good management and financial information and recommended that the *Steering Group on Health Services Information* (the Körner Committee)[14] should examine this. The Körner report on patient transport was issued in 1983.[15] The Naylor recommendations emphasised that communications technology could greatly improve the efficiency of ambulance use. Small control stations have been closed progressively during the last decade in favour of centralised control, although this has not always pleased general practitioners. Ambulance staff need proper training, including advanced training for some staff to equip them for major emergencies. The Naylor recommendations called for more resources to be made available for this training, which is under the broad supervision of the National Staff Committee for ambulance staff, but each authority is responsible for the training of its own staff. Some authorities have grouped together to set up special training schools.

Development of community care and day hospitals will increase the demand upon the ambulance service further. Some authorities fund a hospital car service which acts as a supplementary service and is especially useful for patients who, for instance, may be only slightly incapacitated, but live in an isolated place with no transport of their own and no access to public transport. The 1982 reorganisation made no major changes to the ambulance service and, as with supplies, one DHA usually manages the service on behalf of several others.

The District Management Team

Following the 1974 reorganisation, DMTs were set up to be responsible to the AHA for the management of districts. Although team members could be monitored and coordinated by the Area Team of Officers, they were, as chief officers of the health authority, equal in status. The 1982 reorganisation removed the Area tier and this extended the responsibilities of the DMT in planning matters and collaboration with other authorities. The membership of the DMT remained the same.

Four members of the DMT are appointed: the administrator, nursing officer, treasurer and medical officer. These are full-time paid senior staff of the DHA. The two other members are practising doctors, a consultant and a general practitioner. There is a third in a teaching district, where the Dean of the medical school joins the team. They are elected by their colleagues and the DHA and other members of the DMT have no direct control of these elections although informal discussion will no doubt take place in the DMT as to likely candidates. In some Districts, medical members serve indefinitely, but in others they fill the post for a fixed term. This arrangement is usually preferred if the doctor wishes to combine membership with his clinical work. Both doctors receive extra remuneration for being on the DMT, although in the case of the GP this is likely to go towards the practice funds to cover any extra expenses accrued whilst the GP is away on DMT business.

DMTs, under the general supervision of the DHA, are free to organise their method of working as they see fit. Accordingly, some DMTs meet formally in committee with agenda papers circulated well in advance and with a committee clerk or another administrator present to take minutes. Such DMTs will probably elect one of their number to be chairman. Many DMTs, however, operate in a more informal manner with no one else present unless specifically invited to discuss a particular issue. Such DMTs are unlikely to appoint a chairman, but the administrator may well take on the responsibility of guiding the meeting from topic to topic on an agenda which he or she will have compiled. Meetings are usually held weekly or fortnightly. In some places the full time officers meet without the two elected doctors.

The Royal Commission and more recently the Griffiths Report have been critical of consensus management. Circular HC(80)8 warned DHAs and DMTs that their corporate responsibilities must not blur the individual responsibilities of DMT members for parts of the service.[16] If officers brought problems to the DMT that they should properly sort out as individual heads of service, it would delay the process of management unduly. Griffiths made much of the lack of drive and lowest common denominator effect resulting from consensus management. Those who support this style argue that managing an organisation as complex as a health District requires discussion, even negotiation, before decisions can be made and, more important still, implemented. Members of the team need to get on together for the process to work well. Two highly publicised occasions when teams failed to agree and were effectively disbanded may have fuelled the criticisms.[17]

Each member of the DMT has other responsibilities. These will be discussed in turn.

The District Administrator

There are three main elements of the administrator's role. First he (of 192 District Administrators only 3 in 1984 were women) in the secretary of the DHA and is responsible for managing the Authority's business. At its simplest, this requires him to compile agendas and make appropriate arrangements for DHA meetings. He can also influence how much the members become involved in other matters and can select issues which members are encouraged to pursue. Because of this he is likely to be closer to the chairman than other DMT colleagues.

Secondly, he is responsible for the general coordination of the District. This responsibility is difficult to define, but becomes obvious if it is not done. Although there is considerable variation in the way the District Administrators do this aspect of their work, they tend to take responsibility for gathering matters 'together and for ensuring that objectives are set and achieved. They often act as spokesmen of the Authority to others, including groups of staff, voluntary bodies, local authorities and through the media and at public meetings, to the community at large.

Third, he is responsible for specific functions in the organisation. He is the chief administrator and must ensure that administration throughout the District is carried out in a orderly and effective manner. He does this through his subordinate administrators. He is head of the information service which is now being expanded beyond just medical records to incorporate a much wider range of data and other information. Support services such as catering, laundry, domestic, gardens and works are all accountable to him. The works function, considerably elevated in status under the 1974 reorganisation, lost some of that independence in 1982 with the District Works Officer being made explicitly the subordinate of the District Administrator, although he will also have professional links with his works counterpart at regional level. At District headquarters, the District Administrator is responsible for the staff undertaking service and capital planning and personnel work.

Other staff who do not have an obvious top manager are broadly gathered under the title paramedical. Because they provide services throughout the District they cannot entirely be accommodated within each administrative unit below District level and thus be accountable to the unit administrator. For instance, it is wise to coordinate occupational therapy or dietetics across the District to make best use of scarce resources. A District Therapist may therefore be appointed who is professionally autonomous (see Chapter 10) but managerially reports to either the District Administrator or District Medical Officer as agreed locally. The management of the remedial professions was under continual discussion throughout the 1970s, but the present arrangements seem to work reasonably well where there is a clear distinction between managerial duties and professional responsibilities. This means the District Administrator is in some ways a general manager of other professions, representing their interests in obtaining additional resources. Implementation of the Griffiths proposals may alter this.

The District Treasurer

The District Treasurer's particular responsibility is for accounts, salaries and wages, internal audit and management accountancy. He (there were only two fmale District Treasurers in 1984) advises the DHA on the financial implications of proposals and makes regular budget reports to the authority, although he is seldom a budget holder, this being the responsibility of individual managers. Circular HC(82)3 on *Financial Directives for Health Authorities*[18] made it clear that all officers have a general responsibility for the security and proper use of DHA property and resources, but the treasurer has a particular concern which is also endorsed by the standards of the professional accountancy body to which he belongs.

Allocation of finance is by no means an easy matter, given the fluctuations in local activity and changing government policies. It is the treasurer's duty to endeavour to accommodate these peaks and troughs so that the Authority is not overspent at the end of the year. A more detailed account of the financial arrangements for Districts can be found in Chapter 6.

The District Nursing Officer

The single largest group of staff come under the managerial and professional control of the District Nursing Officer. This means that she or he is responsible not only for the deployment of staff and the cost of that, but also for maintaining standards of patient care. Forty per cent of the DHA funds are allocated to nursing. Her or his span of authority covers general nursing, midwifery, district nursing, health visiting and psychiatric nursing both for the mentally ill and the mentally handicapped. She or he is unlikely to be qualified in all of these specialties, but may have two or three qualifications and in some cases may be a registered tutor. 103 District Nursing Officers are women and 89 are men (1984). Given the overall majority of women in the profession, men hold a disproportionate number of the DNO posts.

Following the *Report of the Committee on the Senior Nursing Staff Structure* (Salmon Report) 1966,[19] nursing was reorganised to take account of the substantial managerial role undertaken by nurses controlling a large work force which has to provide a service day and night. The nursing structure after 1974 was considered by some to be rather over-elaborate and changes in the early 1980s have aimed at concentrating nursing expertise nearer the patient. Accordingly, nursing officers who had been supervisors of ward sisters have been retitled 'clinical nursing managers' and spend more of their time dealing with standards of patient care. The nursing hierarchy now includes directors of nursing services as second-in-line managers to the district nursing officer. They are usually responsible for a particular nursing specialism, such as community nursing or midwifery. These posts are equivalent in status to unit administrators.

District Medical Officer

The duties of the Area Medical Officer and the District Community Physician were combined in 1982 in the new post of District Medical Officer (DMO). The DMO is the doctor in the District who advises the DHA and others on general medical matters and patterns of disease. The post is largely administrative and covers responsibility for the organisation of medical work and community health services. Many DMOs carry out duties for local authorities in occupational and environmental health matters.

Professional Advisory Machinery

It has been a characteristic of the NHS to supplement the management structure with a comprehensive professional advisory system. This operates at all levels from the DHSS downwards. Over time the elaborateness has led to criticism and following the Royal Commission the Chief Medical Officer of the DHSS set up an investigation which reported in 1981. As a result of this, Districts were advised that following the 1982 reorganisation DHAs would have more discretion as to whether to set up professional advisory committees or not.[20] In the event most, if not all Districts, set up District Medical Advisory Committees with membership from hospital, community and family doctors. Such a committee is additional to the Medical Executive Committee which is for consultants and the Local Medical Committee which is for general practitioners. These committees exist in most places, but in the case of the Medical Executive Committee may only be a sub-committee of the District Management Team. Local Medical Committees are not always conterminous with Districts, having been set up to match FPC boundaries. In a few cases a General Practitioner Committee equivalent in status to the Medical Executive Committee has been set up. Many authorities have also set up District Dental Advisory Committees and Nursing and Midwifery Advisory Committees, although this committee might appear somewhat redundant as the authority already has a chief officer heading the nursing service.

Unit Management

This discussion of the work of the Districts is completed with the management arrangements below District. Under the 1974 reorganisation, sectors were set up to sub-divide the District in a manner which took account of both functional and geographical considerations. Most Districts were too large to be managed effectively on a day-to-day basis from the central headquarters. Sector administrators succeeded hospital secretaries and divisional nursing officers replaced the matrons of pre-Salmon Report days. In the 1982 reorganisation based on *Patients First*, decision-making responsibility was to be at the lowest reasonable level, so unit teams were set up with a unit administrator, a director of nursing services and a doctor. They were made responsible for the management of the unit, mirroring in some ways the corporate style of the DMT. However, there are important differences. The administrator and the nurse were subordinates of DMT officers and it is possible that unit corporate decisions might conflict with those taken by the chief officers at District. For instance the unit team might wish to transfer the money from unfilled nursing posts to paramedical staff, only to find that the District Nursing Officer would prefer to use that money to transfer resources away from that unit to another, for instance from an acute unit to the community. Another difference centres on what best constitutes a unit. Circular HC(80)8 gave five possibilities, some favouring a geographical entity, others reflecting a common task. Should psychiatry be organised on a unit basis even if the care is provided in four hospitals many miles apart, two of which also look after patients in other specialties? Deciding on the best arguments locally has inevitably involved compromise.

In the planning process, units were encouraged to put forward new ideas and ways of managing the services within the context of District guidelines. Budgetary control cannot be fully developed to unit level. Not all budget holders worked within one unit, particularly specialist staff such as speech therapists or dietitians. Despite these practical points, most unit teams found a way of working which enhanced the quality of management within the District and involved consultants and general practitioners. The Griffiths Report proposed the appointment of a general manager at unit level and this will influence any reorganisation of working style that is introduced.

Conclusion

A short time after the 1982 reorganisation the District concept is firmly established and authority members and officers show more enthusiasm than at the same time after the 1974 reorganisation. This may be in part because the framework is not now so unfamiliar as it was then and because it gives more weight to practical considerations such as natural communities and catchment areas of a district general hospital.

Notes

1. DHSS Circular HC(80)8. *Health Service Development Structure and Management*, July, 1980.
2. Ibid., para. 2.
3. DHSS Circular HC(81)6. *Health Services Management Membership of District Health Authorities*, May, 1981.
4. Circular HC(80)9. Op. cit., para. 10.
5. DHSS. *Democracy in the National Health Service: Membership of Health Authorities*, HMSO, London, 1974.
6. Circular HC(81)6. Op. cit.
7. Dr Christopher Ham is undertaking a study of health authority members in Croydon and Bath. His preliminary work is described in *Health and Social Services Journal*, p. 222, 23 February, 1984.
8. House of Commons. Parliamentary Debates. Official Report. *Hansard*, 20 December 1983, p. 298. The Secretary of State speaking at the second reading of the Health and Social Security Bill said: 'Under the new arrangements (proposed in the Bill) we shall have a single line of authority between family practitioner committees and the Secretaries of State. FPCs will become employing authorities in their own right, they will be responsible for their own services, and they will be answerable for their own management costs. I believe that this will improve not only their accountability but administrative efficiency . . .'
9. Central Health Services Council. *Final Report of the Committee on Hospital Supplies* (Messer Report), HMSO, London, 1958.
10. Ministry of Health. *Report of the Committee on Hospital Supplies Organisation* (Hunt Report), HMSO, 1966.

11. DHSS. *Regional Chairmen's Enquiry into the Working of the DHSS in relation to Regional Health Authorities* (Three Chairmen's Report), 1976.

12. DHSS. *Buying for the National Health Service* (Collier Report), HMSO, 1976.

13. DHSS. *Report of the Supply Board Working Group* (Salmon Report), HMSO, London, 1978.

14. DHSS. *Steering Group on Health Services Information* (Chaired by Edith Körner), 1982 onwards.

15. The Körner Working Group G produced an interim report on patient transport services in January, 1983.

16. Circular (80)8. Op. cit., para. 24.

17. In Solihull, Birmingham, the DMT could not agree and were replaced although three of the officers subsequently found other chief officer posts.

18. DHSS Circular HC(82)3. *Financial Directives for Health Authorities in England*, February, 1982.

19. Ministry of Health and SHHD. *Report of the Committee on Senior Nursing Staff Structure* (Salmon Report), HMSO, London, 1966.

20. DHSS Circular HC(82). *Health Service Development: Professional Advisory Machinery*, January, 1982.

5 THE NHS IN SCOTLAND, WALES AND NORTHERN IRELAND

Introduction

Because the general principles governing the NHS are the same throughout the United Kingdom, it is easy to assume that the way health services are organised in Wales, Scotland and Northern Ireland is the same as in England. This is not the case. This chapter outlines the more important variations between the four countries, with particular emphasis on Scotland.

Scotland

1 April 1974 was the appointed day for the reorganisation of the NHS in Scotland as it was in England and Wales. The legislation that originally created the Scottish Health Service was the National Health Service (Scotland) Act, 1947, passed on 21 May 1947, and it established an organisation based on the same tripartite principle as in England and Wales. The hospital and specialist services were administered by five Regional Hospital Boards: Northern, North-Eastern, Eastern, South-Eastern and Western with sixty-five Boards of Management between them, analogous to the Hospital Management Committees in England and Wales. Family practitioner services were administered by twenty-five executive councils, and there were fifty-five local health authorities providing community and environmental health services. The Secretary of State for Scotland was responsible for the whole of the NHS in Scotland, with support from civil servants in the Scottish Home and Health Department.

In December 1968, after extensive consultations with a wide range of interested parties both within and outside the NHS, the Secretary of State for Scotland published a Green Paper containing suggestions for reorganising the service called *Administrative Reorganisation of the Scottish Health Services*.[1] It met with a wide measure of support which enabled the Secretary of State to proceed with the publication of a White Paper in July 1971 entitled *Reorganisation of the Scottish Health Services*[2] containing the government's proposals for legislation to

Figure 6 *Scottish Health Boards*

AREA	AREA POPULATION	NO. OF DISTRICTS PER AREA					TEACHING DISTRICTS	DISTRICT POPULATIONS (000s)			
		1	2	3	4	5		< 50	50–149	150–249	250+
Argyll and Clyde	456000				*		—		3	1	
Ayrshire and Arran	367000		*				—			2	
Borders	99000	*					—		1		
Dumfries and Galloway	144000	*					—		1		
Fife	328000		*				—		1	1	
Forth Valley	263000		*				—		2		
Grampian	436000			*			1		2	1	
Greater Glasgow	1126000					*	5			2	3
Highlands	175000		*				—	1	1		
Lanarkshire	610000			*			—			3	
Lothian	742000			*			2		1		2
Orkney	17000	*					—	1			
Shetland	18000	*					—	1			
Tayside	397000			*			1		2	1	
Western Isles	31000	*					—	1			
	5229000	5	4	4	1	1	9	4	14	11	5

Source: SHHD Circular HSR(73)C31

institute the reorganisation. The *National Health Service (Scotland) Bill* was introduced in Parliament in January 1972 and received Royal Assent on 9 August 1972. There remained just under two years for preparation to be made to implement the new arrangements. No specific study was commissioned to analyse the management arrangements in the new structure, although the Grey Book (published by the DHSS) did not apply to Scotland. However, the Scottish Home and Health Department started a new series of circulars giving guidance to the health authorities (HSR Series − Health Service Reorganisation Scotland) and the Information Office of the Scottish Office was also very active in disseminating information to bodies within and outside the NHS.

Under the National Health Service (Scotland) Act, 1972, health boards were created for each area of Scotland to act as the single authority for administering the three branches of the former tripartite structure. The Scottish National Health Service Staff Commission was consulted on the handling of the recruiting, transferring and appointing of staff before and during the period of reorganisation, and the reviewing of the arrangements so that the interests of the 100,000 affected staff would be safeguarded. Two new bodies without precedents in the pre-1974 structure were created at national level − the Scottish Health Service Planning Council and the Common Services Agency. These are not precisely mirrored in England, their functions being shared by the DHSS and the Regional Health Authorities, although in Wales, the Welsh Health Technical Services Organisation shares some features of the Scottish Common Services Agency. Provision was made for professional advice to be available both nationally and locally through consultative committees, but no specific bodies were established to pursue collaboration between the local and health authorities in the same way as the Joint Consultative Committees in England and Wales. There was, however, provision for health boards with higher populations to set up administrative organisations in districts to handle some of their functions locally (see Figure 6) There are bodies for representing the views of users of the health services in each district or undivided area called Local Health Councils (see Figure 7). The 1972 Act also established the Health Service Commissioner for Scotland who started work on 1 October 1973, and is currently the same individual as the Commissioner for England and Wales, and the Parliamentary Commissioner (the Ombudsman).

The reorganisation of local government created new local authorities in Scotland which came into being on 15 May 1975 − that is, just over

Figure 7 *Organisation of the Scottish NHS*

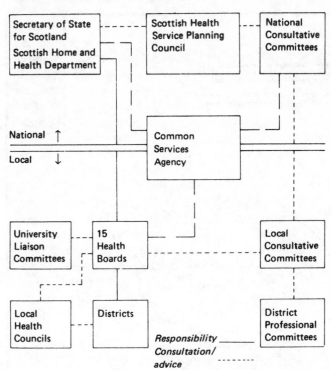

Source: Scottish Information Office

a year after the NHS reorganisation and the new local authorities in England and Wales. There were nine Regional authorities divided into fifty-six Districts, and three Island Councils created by the Local Government (Scotland) Act, 1973, and their boundaries closely followed the health board boundaries, the main difference being that the Strathclyde Region contained four health boards. This Act also provided for local community councils within the Districts – a feature absent from the arrangements in England and Wales.

Health Boards

The fifteen health boards in Scotland were directly responsible to the

Figure 8 *Scottish Health Board Boundaries*

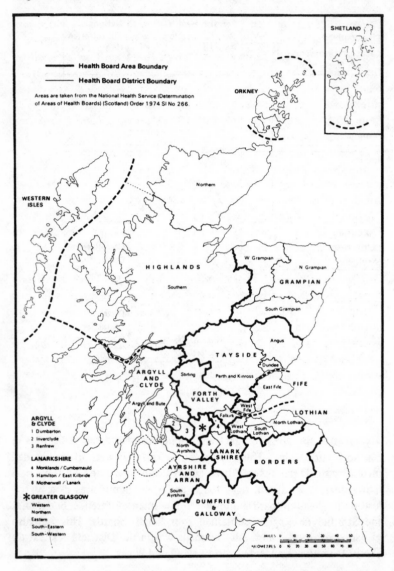

Source: Scottish Office Brief on the National Health Service in Scotland, 1974

Secretary of State for Scotland for the planning and provision of integrated health services in their areas. Figure 8 shows the area boundaries, and indicates how ten of the fifteen areas were divided into Districts. Each board had a chairman appointed by the Secretary of State and between fourteen and twenty-two members appointed from nominations put forward by regional and district local government authorities, trades unions, the health care professions, the universities and a variety of other organisations. In July 1974 the Secretary of State issued a discussion paper called *The National Health Service and the Community in Scotland*.[3]

The health boards as such were concerned mainly with major policy matters and the broad allocation of resources, delegating authority to manage the service to four senior officers of the board — the Chief Administrative Medical Officer, the Chief Area Nursing Officer, the Treasurer and the Secretary — who together constituted the Area Executive Group. These officers had both individual professional and team responsibilities in a similar way to the Area Team of Officers of the AHAs in England and Wales. The Chief Administrative Dental Officer and the Chief Pharmacist joined the Area Executive Group for the discussion of items relevant to their responsibilities. The team had to present advice and information to the board to help it to establish policy and priorities. Day-to-day management in the larger Boards which were divided into Districts is referred to below. Health boards were encouraged to set up area programme planning committees, similar to the English district health care planning teams. Most boards created such committees for the main groups of users.

Family Practitioner Services

There is no separate administration of family practitioners' contracts in Scotland to compare with the FPCs in England and Wales. General medical and dental practitioners, pharmacists and opticians hold contracts directly with the health boards, who also arrange for all the necessary paymaster, registration and service committee functions. This is a notable step towards integration which has not been achieved in England and Wales and indeed the 1984 legislation will make it less likely (see Chapter 4).

University Liaison

Collaboration in varying degrees between the universities with medical schools and the health boards was formalised through the establishment of four University Liaison Committees one for each of the universities with medical and dental schools. At least one third of the membership was nominated by the universities having an interest in the health services in the Area, an equal number were nominated by the health board (or boards) and there were some other members. The University Liaison Committees are the descendants of the Medical Education Committees set up under the 1947 Act which advised the Regional Hospital Boards on clinical teaching and research provision.

District Organisation

In each of the Districts, there were four officers directly responsible to their counterparts on the Area Executive Group, but they had a considerable degree of independence. The District Administrator, District Nursing Officer, District Medical Officer and the District Finance Officer constituted the District Executive Group, and they were, as such, jointly accountable to the Area Executive Group for a number of functions. An important difference between the District organisations in Scotland and in England and Wales was therefore that the Scottish District Officers were directly subordinate to their Area Officers although both are officers of the health board. The relationship in England and Wales was described in terms of monitoring and co-ordinating rather than as direct line responsibility, with a view to ensuring that the District organisation was not placed in a subordinate position. Another important difference is that in Scotland there are no GP or hospital consultant representatives directly involved in the District management arrangements.[4] This is because there has always been a much stronger tradition of medical administration in Scotland. Before 1934 medical superintendents had not dwindled as they had done south of the border. Clinicians are used to working with administrative medical colleagues. Community physicians are also often found on unit management teams.

Further Reorganisation

The criticism regarding too many levels of management was not appropriate to Scotland where health boards in some respects undertook both the Regional and Area role. *Patients First* only applied to England and Wales but a similar document was issued for Scotland suggesting that health boards review their administrative structures with a view to simplifying them. A reduction in functional management and more devolution to Units was also suggested. This review was to be undertaken and changes made by the date of the English reorganisation, 1 April 1982. In the event reorganisation in Scotland has taken much longer. Only ten of the health boards had subordinate Districts. Glasgow and Lothian were very large. For instance, the Greater Glasgow Health Board administered 14,500 beds, 32,000 staff and a budget of £330 million (1982 figures) to serve a population of 1.2 million. Lothian's 1982 budget was £250 million. Both these Boards were therefore much larger than any District in England. The Highland Board however with a relatively small population covered an enormous area so that some sort of sub-division seemed desirable. Lanarkshire and Tayside also wished to keep a District structure. Late in the day Argyll and Clyde having first opted in favour of a single District changed its mind. Difficulties arose from the inability of the Whitley Councils and others to agree on the appropriate grades for posts in the new structure, particularly those at Unit level when many of the units were as large as English Districts. Somewhat suddenly and apparently disregarding much restructuring work that some health boards had done, the Secretary of State for Scotland announced on 10th November 1983 that all Districts would be scrapped leaving health boards with subordinate Units only. In the spirit of the Griffiths report (which had not considered Scotland or Northern Ireland) it was felt a simpler organisation would improve management. The gross disparity in Unit size seems likely to lead to problems and there has been some evidence of migration of chief officers to England to avoid these difficulties.

Local Health Councils

It is the responsibility of each health board to establish local health councils (similar to community health councils in England and Wales) normally for each district. Their membership, which ranges from totals of eighteen to thirty, is drawn from the local authorities, voluntary organisations, trade unions and other local bodies, the normal term of appointment being for four years, half the membership retiring every two years. Each local health council produces an annual report which is submitted to the health board, and copies go to the Secretary of State.

Initially, the process of establishment was delayed, and the first of the forty-eight local health councils did not meet until March 1975. The discussion paper published in July 1974 suggested that the formation of a National Association of Local Health Councils, could, among other functions, provide nominations to the Scottish Health Service Planning Council, and it raised the possibility of giving LHCs the right to nominate two of their members to their health board. The National Association of LHCs was set up in 1977.

Central Organisation

The Secretary of State for Scotland is, through the form of the NHS legislation, personally accountable to Parliament for the Scottish health services in the same way as the Secretary of State for Social Services and the Secretary of State for Wales are for the NHS in England and Wales. In Scotland, the supreme government department is the Scottish Office, and Figure 9 shows how the Ministers' responsibilities are arranged. The senior civil servant in the Scottish Office is the Permanent Under-Secretary of State, and he presides over the Management Group which includes the senior civil servants from the five other major government departments in Scotland.

Scottish Home and Health Department

The department responsible to the Secretary of State for the central administration of the Scottish NHS is the Scottish Home and Health Department (SHHD). This department is also responsible for the central administration relating to the police service, criminal justice, legal aid, the administration of prisons, the administration and legislation relating to superannuation of public service employees, the organisation of the fire service, home defence and emergency services, the legislation relating to shops, theatres and cinemas, licensed premises and land tenure matters.

Within the SHHD there are a number of officers of the health professions including the Chief Medical Officer for Scotland and his staff of Medical Officers, the Chief Dental Officer and his staff, the Chief Pharmacist, and the Chief Nursing Officer and her staff. Together with senior departmental officials, the chief officers form the policy group. The SHHD has been reorganised to reflect the changed administrative structure of the NHS, and four Divisions within it are responsible for central plans and policy in relation to health care, while five other Divisions are responsible for different aspects of the use of resources.

Figure 9 *Scottish Government Departments*

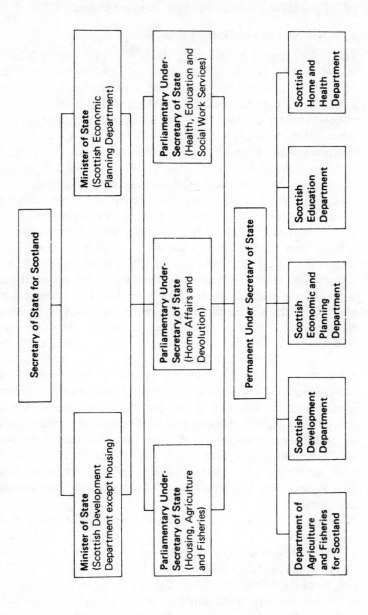

Scottish Health Service Planning Council

This body, created by the 1972 Act, was partly derived from the former Scottish Health Services Council, an influential body which advised the Secretary of State on the shaping of policy for health service provision in Scotland. Like the Central Health Services Council, its counterpart in England and Wales, it was made up of representatives from all the major professional groups with an interest in the health services. The new Planning Council was created to ensure that effective strategies could be devised and implemented to improve Scottish health service provision on an integrated basis, in a context of limited available resources, with the fullest participation from the health authorities. The membership therefore specifically includes one representative from each health board, one from each university with a medical school, six officers from the SHHD and some other members appointed by the Secretary of State, as is the independent chairman of this Planning Council. Just as the DHSS has to work closely with the regional health authorities in England and with the Welsh Office to secure effective planning, so the Scottish Planning Council has to ensure comprehensive targets can be established, and that progress towards their achievement is carefully monitored. A number of programme planning committees have been set up with members of the Council and specialists nominated by the eight national consultative committees of the various health professions. The Council gives advice on the implementation of agreed policies and on evaluation of the success of the policies. A policy group of top Scottish Home and Health Department officials is linked to the Planning Council by the Planning Unit of officials. For instance the Council prepared a report which was published in December 1980 with the Secretary of State's blessing entitled *Priorities for Health Care in Scotland*. The report allocated services into three categories as follows.

Category A – Expenditure to grow faster than overall expenditure
  Prevention
  Services for the multiply deprived
  Community nursing services
  Care of the elderly
  Elderly with mental disability
  Mental illness
  Mental handicap
  Physical handicap

Category B – Expenditure to grow but at a slower rate than Category A
  Primary dental services

Maternity services
General medical services
General ophthalmic services
Category C — Expenditure to remain static or to decline
Child health services
Acute hospital services
General pharmaceutical services

Common Services Agency

With the requirements that the health boards should administer their services on an integrated basis, and with the disappearance of the Regional Hospital Boards, a central mechanism was sought for providing supporting services so that health boards would not have to duplicate these functions unnecessarily and uneconomically. The Common Services Agency (CSA) was therefore established to run those services that could be organised centrally in this way. Figure 10 sets out the main functions of the CSA — many of the 6,000 staff involved in providing them were previously doing similar work, but were either directly employed by the SHHD, the Regional Hospital Boards or Executive Councils. The CSA is therefore a loose federation of agencies each providing different services, under the supervision of a Management Committee. The Chairman is a health board chairman, and three members are health board members, three members are health board officers and five members are SHHD officers, all being appointed by the Secretary of State.

Medical Services

Scotland has for centuries maintained a strong tradition of medical education to very high standards, and its four university medical schools (Edinburgh, Glasgow, Aberdeen and Dundee) produce one fifth of all medical graduates in the United Kingdom. The professional bodies have grown up independently of those in England and have achieved notable prominence. The Royal College of Physicians (Edinburgh), the Royal College of Surgeons (Edinburgh) and the Royal College of Physicians and Surgeons (Glasgow) are the oldest; the Scottish Radiological Society, the Scottish Committee for Community Medicine and Scottish members of the Royal Colleges of General Practitioners, Obstetricians and Gynaecologists and Pathologists, the Faculties of Anaesthetists and of Community Medicine join them in

Figure 10 *Common Services Agency*

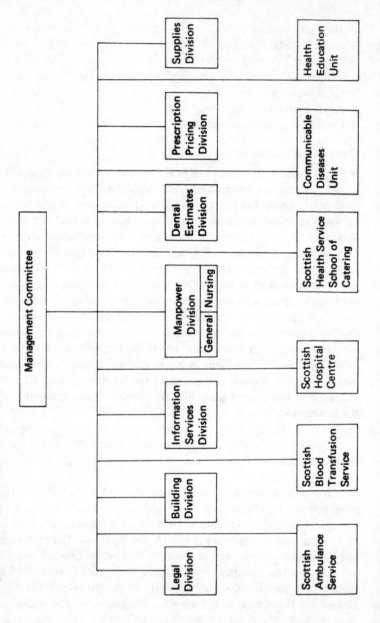

being recognised professional groups contributing advice through the National Medical Consultative Committee to the Planning Council. The BMA is also active in Scotland and its Scottish General Medical Services Committee contributes to the National Medical Consultative Committee. The Scottish Junior Staffs Group Council is a similar body to the Hospital Junior Staffs Group Council for England and Wales, while hospital consultants are represented through the Scottish Committee for Hospital Medical Services. In the field of postgraduate medicine, the Scottish Council for Postgraduate Medical Education was founded in May 1970 to promote the ongoing development of medical practitioners through extensive programmes of teaching and refresher courses.

Health centres are a more prominent feature of health care in Scotland than in England and Wales, and the SHHD has been pursuing a policy which is designed to provide extra health care for 50 per cent of the total population (about 5.3 million) from health centres by 1980, and for 80 per cent by 1985. In fact this seems unlikely to be achieved as by the end of 1983 there were 168 health centres involving 1,127 GPs, which represented 36 per cent of all GPs.[4] This number is higher than in England. Two particularly interesting schemes, in Woodside (Glasgow) and Clydebank, each involve up to thirty GPs in providing care for populations as large as 70,000. Two further large health centres are planned for Dumbarton and East Kilbride. Over 50 per cent of GPs practise in groups of two or three, and the average list size is 2,000 patients. Links with the hospital service are strong, and 400 GPs hold hospital specialist appointments, while 300 GPs have access to beds in community hospitals.

Major hospital redevelopment has taken place in Scotland in the last fifteen years starting with Ninewells Hospital, Dundee, and Victoria Hospital, Kirkcaldy.

There are a number of other professional and administrative bodies with important duties in the Scottish National Health Service which are similar in constitutions and objectives to those bodies described in the chapters relating to England and Wales. These include the Scottish Hospital Advisory Service, the Scottish Medical Practices Committee, the Scottish Tribunal, the Mental Welfare Commission and the Scottish National Board for Nurses. In addition, the mental health services are governed by the provisions of the Mental Health (Scotland) Act, 1966, and social work probation and after care services are covered by the Social Work (Scotland) Act, 1968.

Wales

The laws of Wales are generally much closer to England's than those of Scotland or Northern Ireland. Arrangements for health care are similarly more alike, but organisationally there are differences. Up to 1974 there was a Welsh Hospital Board, local health authorities and executive councils as in England. Thereafter, the Welsh Office was allocated both Departmental and Regional responsibilities with a Health and Social Services Department under the overall responsibility of the Secretary of State for Wales. This minister is responsible to the Parliament in Westminster for a variety of functions in addition to health. This variety of responsibilities has led to periodic criticisms: the Royal Commission noted in 1979 that the Welsh Office was too remote from health authorities and their problems.[5] However, a Regional Authority as well as the Area tier would have been excessive, given that the whole population of Wales is only 2.7 million (which is similar to that of a smallish Region in England). The heavy industrialised area of South Wales separated by mountains and relatively poor road and rail services from the rest of the country, has always made communication difficult.

In 1974 eight Area Health Authorities were set up which were conterminous with county councils (see Figure 11). Three of these were single District areas, three had two Districts and two had four Districts. Unlike England, the District officers were made subordinate to their Area counterparts. Wales, like England, had Community Health Councils and Family Practitioner Committees, but unlike England, Wales set up a common services agency known as the Welsh Health Technical Services Organisation (WHTSO) (see Figure 12). This organisation remained after the 1982 changes. It does not have managerial authority over the Area Health Authorities (pre-1982) or the District Health Authorities (since 1982), but it carries out tasks on behalf of these authorities and for the Welsh Office. Its main areas of activity are: building services, management services, supplies, prescription pricing, computer organisation and some other miscellaneous administrative services. The small board running WHTSO is appointed by, and is responsible to, the Secretary of State for Wales and there are designated senior officers for each area of activity.

Patients First asserted that there needed to be a general change in structure in Wales and that there should be some re-drawing of boundaries.[6] But this superficial observation needed more backing so a more lengthy consultative document[7] was issued by the Secretary of State

Figure 11 *Welsh Health District Boundaries*

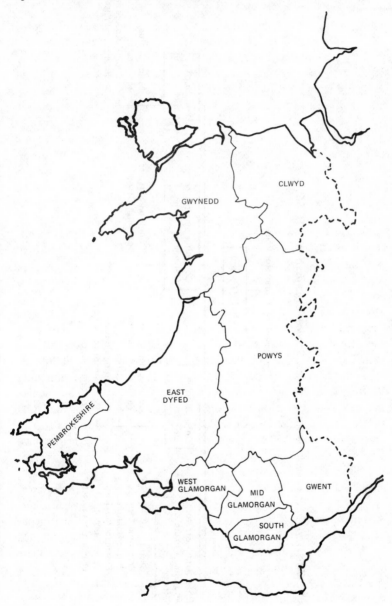

Source: Hospitals and Health Services Yearbook ISHA, 1983.

Figure 12 *The Work of the Welsh Health Technical Services Organisation (WHTSO)*

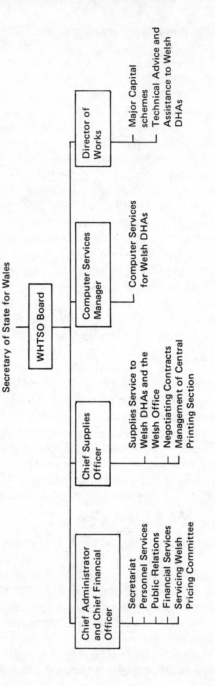

Secretary of State for Wales

WHTSO Board

Chief Administrator and Chief Financial Officer
- Secretariat
- Personnel Services
- Public Relations
- Financial Services
- Servicing Welsh Pricing Committee

Chief Supplies Officer
- Supplies Service to Welsh DHAs and the Welsh Office
- Negotiating Contracts
- Management of Central Printing Section

Computer Services Manager
- Computer Services for Welsh DHAs

Director of Works
- Major Capital schemes
- Technical Advice and Assistance to Welsh DHAs

for Wales asking for opinions on a variety of matters including the removal of Districts, the splitting of Dyfed and Mid-Glamorgan authorities and the setting-up of a coordinating all-Wales body to be called the Welsh Health Council. Following consultation, the official position was amended so that Areas were to become Districts. Dyfed was to be split into two health authorities, Pembrokeshire and East Dyfed. Mid-Glamorgan, however, was to be retained, but with strengthened management. Finally, there was not to be a Welsh Health Council, as this proposal has excited little support. The appointed day was the same as in England, 1 April 1982, but the titles of some of the chief officers were different. For instance the District Nursing Officer (or sometimes Chief Nursing Officer in England) is now called the Chief Administrative Nursing Officer in Wales.

The Griffiths Report referred to England only, but in December 1983 the Secretary of State for Wales issued a letter inviting comments on the Griffiths proposal.[8] Significantly, this letter, by inviting DHAs to identify general managers there and then, went further than the letter issued three weeks earlier in England. In one case, this was interpreted as giving the go-ahead to make the appointment immediately. The letter also referred to the need to strengthen the managerial functions of the Welsh Office and this reflected the criticism found by the Royal Commission five years previously that the Welsh Office was too remote. A Health Policy Board with a subordinate Executive Committee were proposed to mirror the functions of the Griffiths supervisory and managerial boards at DHSS level. The idea of a Welsh Health Council, therefore, returned in a slightly different guise. Meanwhile the All-Wales Health Forum is occasionally called by the Secretary of State for Wales to discuss major issues such as mental handicap strategy or future management arrangements after the Griffiths report. This group is broadly representative but has no statutory responsibility.

Northern Ireland

The organisation of health care in Northern Ireland differs most from England. This reflects different traditions and the unstable political structure of the country. During the last half-century, Northern Ireland has sometimes exercised considerable autonomy with its own parliament at Stormont, but recently has been subject to direct rule from London. The first reorganisation of the health service took place slightly earlier than in England, with legislation passed in 1972 being implemented in October 1973.[9] From that day the Province was organised into four Health and Social Services Boards (see Figure 13) who were accountable to the Secretary of State for Northern Ireland, and whose chairmen and vice chairmen were, and still are, appointed directly by him. The Boards had a mixed membership: thirty per cent of whom were district council nominees, thirty per cent were from the professions and the remainder from voluntary bodies and other lay bodies. The Boards were geographical as their names suggest; Eastern, Northern, Western and Southern were responsible for seventeen Districts covering populations from 43,300 in Omagh to 250,000 in North and West Belfast. The total population of Northern Ireland is 1.5 million. The Districts were roughly conterminous with local authority district councils, but these bodies have fewer responsibilities than their counterparts in England. For instance, education and library services are run centrally for all Northern Ireland and housing, an important policy area, is managed by the Northern Ireland Housing Executive operating through its own regional offices. As health and social services are run by one administration the need for the English style joint planning and joint financing arrangements is much reduced. Statutory responsibilities are not always the same as in England. For instance, the education of the mentally handicapped remains with the Health and Social Services Board in Northern Ireland, whereas in England it was transferred to education authorities in 1972.

As in Scotland and Wales, certain functions are not provided by the Health and Social Services Board directly, but are undertaken centrally through the Central Services Agency. In Northern Ireland this body does work which in England is the responsibility of the Family Practitioner Committees. The Agency is also responsible for prescription pricing, for certain personnel duties concerning hospital doctors down to registrar level, for supplies, support services, advice and legal matters. Consumer interests in Northern Ireland are represented by District Committees, operating in a manner similar to the English CHCs.

Area Boards, which were described as being responsible for administering, planning, monitoring and coordinating health and social services within their Areas to help them form committees, were set up. The Policy and Resources Committee was responsible for matching capital and revenue allocations to the needs and demands of the service after consultation with professional and managerial staff within the Area and its subordinate Districts (after 1983, Units). The Health Services Committee and the Personal Social Services Committee were responsible

Figure 13 *Northern Ireland Health and Social Services Boundaries*

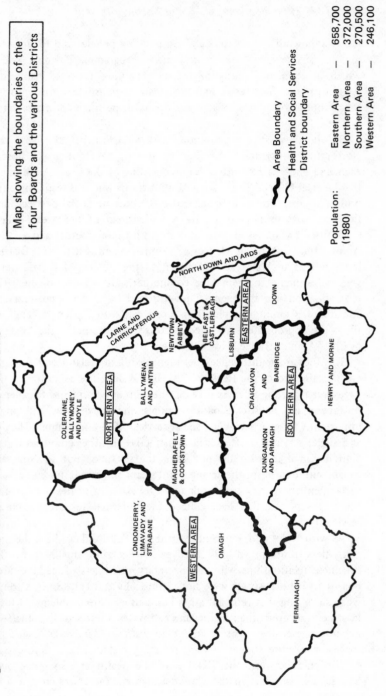

Map showing the boundaries of the four Boards and the various Districts

— Area Boundary

Health and Social Services District boundary

Population: (1980)

Eastern Area	—	658,700
Northern Area	—	372,000
Southern Area	—	270,500
Western Area	—	246,100

for recommending objectives and formulating policies and for improving the service having taken account of Programme Planning Teams which are similar to English District Planning Teams. Finally, the Administrative Services Committee had responsibility for ensuring that proper procedures existed for financial, personnel and associated matters.

Before the last reorganisation in 1983 (Western, Southern and Northern Boards) and 1984 (Eastern Board), the four health boards each had an Area Executive Team consisting of the Chief Administrative Medical Officer, Chief Area Administrator who was responsible for both administration and finance, the Director of Social Services, and the team was usually joined by the Chairman of the Area Medical Committee (who was almost invariably a hospital doctor) and a Chief Administrative Nursing Officer. A similar team existed at District level, but as in Wales and Scotland, all the officers at District level were subordinate to their Area counterparts. A criticism of the 1973 reorganisation was that general practitioners had little opportunity to contribute. Community physician posts had often been difficult to fill as the appropriately qualified doctors tended to prefer the Area job of Chief Administrative Medical Officer.

The four main differences between Northern Ireland and England are the absence of the Regional tier (like Wales), the exclusion of the Treasurer from the Executive Team, the joint appointment of academic posts working in Area Board hospitals and universities and, most importantly, the inclusion of social services. The combining of health and social services is often seen as attractive to other countries in the United Kingdom who do not have that system. But in Northern Ireland enthusiasm for the arrangement seems somewhat muted because each member of the team tends to be loyal to his or her own professional group and this has reduced the potential for integration of services.

As with Wales and Scotland, Northern Ireland did not have the too-many-tiers problem in 1982. Given the relative smallness of the Province, relationships with the Secretary of State's office, the Area boards and the Districts were not intrinsically difficult. So it is somewhat surprising that reorganisation has caused more problems, at least in structural terms, than in England and Wales if not Scotland. In 1979 a consultative document[10] similar to *Patients First* was issued. It suggested a more straightforward planning system and a clarification of the role between the DHSS and the health and social services boards. As elsewhere in the United Kingdom, there was considerable emphasis on the simplification of administration and the proposal was made that Districts should be abolished although the difference in size between the Eastern Board and those elsewhere in the Province was thought to be a difficulty as indeed it proved to be. The membership of teams was reviewed and as well as the addition of the GP, it was proposed that the finance officer become a full member of the team, echoing the advice of the Royal Commission on the management of financial resources in the NHS[11] issued in 1978. This has not happened.

In July 1980, the Secretary of State issued a statement asking for more consultation, but indicating his intention that the four health and social services boards should remain, that Districts should be disbanded and in their stead Units set up supported by Unit Management Groups, but without the corporate status that District Executive Teams had had. These proposals were confirmed in circular HSS(P)1/81 *The Structure and Management of Health and Personal Social Services in Northern Ireland* issued in June 1981. The detailed arrangements were set out in circular HSS(P)183 which listed the objectives of the restructuring as:

(i)   to ensure better (i.e. more effective and more economical) planning and management arrangements which would improve services to patients and clients;

(ii) to free Boards and their Chief Officers from undue involvement in decisions on day-to-day management, so as to allow them to concentrate on major issues of policy, planning, resources allocation and monitoring of services;

(iii) to secure delegation of day-to-day management decisions to officials at the operational level or point of delivery of services with (save in the most exceptional circumstances) no intermediate tier of management between them and Chief Officers at area level;

(iv) to reduce the cost of administration to the minimum compatible with the efficient management and use of resources;

(v)   to further the integrated planning and delivery of health and personal social services and of hospital and community care;

(vi) to clarify relationships between the Department and Boards and between the Boards and the Central Services Agency and the Staff Council; and

(vii) to clarify roles and responsibilities of staff within Boards at both area and operational levels.

The new structure was meant to have been implemented on 1 April 1982 with the possible exception of the Eastern Board. Further discussions delayed the changes and the reorganisation of the other three boards formally started on 1 April 1983. The position of Belfast in the Eastern Board, as of Glasgow and for similar reasons, became more confused as discussions on the number of Units increased. There had been six Districts previously, but now 14 Units were proposed. A proposal by the Northern Ireland Assembly that the board should be replaced by two boards was rejected by the Parliamentary Under Secretary of State for Northern Ireland. Instead, the new board would have two committees, an Administrative Services Committee and a Policy and Resources Committee. This might seem to be introducing a tier of management between Units and the board itself. As a result, implementation of the changes was expected to be delayed further. Unlike in England, these changes were not popular, particularly with the chief officers who could find themselves downgraded from their District Chief Officer posts to lower status at Unit level.

Conclusion

The differences in organisations of the health service in the four countries comprising the United Kingdom may seem somewhat unnecessary. They are certainly confusing to professionals who work in more than one of these countries. Nevertheless, they arise from the different legal and political traditions of each country. They also reflect demographic and geographical differences. A fuller analysis would give detailed comparisons of health statistics which would provide a basis for assessing the effectiveness of the health service. For instance, although Scotland has more doctors per head of population than the rest of the United Kingdom, the expectation of life is two or three years less. Such a statistic means little on its own and would have to be developed against various other health and performance indicators to have any particular significance. As will be seen in Chapter 13, comparisons with other countries help to judge how effective the health service is. Comparisons within the NHS also show that despite the achievements of the first 35 years, fundamental differences in patient care still exist within the United Kingdom itself.

Notes

1. Scottish Home and Health Department. *Administrative Reorganisation of the Scottish Health Services*, HMSO, Edinburgh, 1968.

2. Scottish Home and Health Department. *Reorganisation of the Scottish Health Services*, HMSO, Edinburgh, 1971 (Cmnd 4734).

3. Scottish Home and Health Department. *The National Health Service and the Community in Scotland*, HMSO, Edinburgh, 1970.

4. Scottish Health Boards Returns 1983.

5. Royal Commission on the National Health Service, p. 305, para. 19.25, HMSO, London, 1979 (Cmnd 7615).

6. DHSS. *Patients First*, paras. 46 and 47, HMSO, London, 1979.

7. Welsh Office. *The Structure and Management of the NHS in Wales*, HMSO, Cardiff, 1980.

8. Welsh Office. *The NHS Management Inquiry, Implementation in Wales*, letter dated 13th December 1983.

9. *The Health and Personal Social Services (HI) Order 1972.*

10. DHSS. *Consultative Paper on the Structure and Management of Health and Personal Social Services in Northern Ireland*, HMSO, Belfast, December 1979.

11. *Report of the Royal Commission on the National Health Service on the Management of Financial Resources in the National Health Service with particular reference to Northern Ireland*, HMSO, London, 1978.

6 FINANCING THE NATIONAL HEALTH SERVICE

This chapter is concerned with three basic questions: what does it cost to run the NHS? where does the money to pay for the service come from? what are the implications of this system?

Capital and Revenue Expenditure

Traditionally, NHS expenditure is divided into two categories — capital and revenue. Capital expenditure is the purchase cost of an asset which generates benefits over more than one year. Examples of such assets in the NHS include the purchase of land for building, the erection of new buildings, the extension of old buildings and the adaptation of existing buildings for health purposes, and the cost of initial equipment, furniture and stores for these buildings. These costs are incurred in relation to hospitals, clinics, health centres and for offices of administrative bodies such as the health authorities themselves. Revenue expenditure, on the other hand, covers the costs of services and assets which generate in the current year. These include the remuneration of medical, nursing, paramedical and other professional staff; the remuneration of administrators, accountants, storekeepers, cooks, domestics, porters, engineers and maintenance staff; the cost of goods and services needed to provide residential care for patients and accommodation for staff; the cost of drugs, appliances, fuel and the replacement of equipment and maintenance of buildings. These lists of items are not exhaustive but simply indicate how the whole range of health service costs have been classified.

The reason for making a distinction between NHS capital and revenue expenditure may not immediately be clear, since in private industry it is essential for the calculation of the annual profit margin. Profit is the income derived from a given level of expenditure, and this calculation is obviously difficult to transfer to the accounts of the NHS, where the 'income' is not represented in monetary terms. There are, however, four reasons why the capital/revenue distinction is made in the financing of the NHS.

First, a decision on spending priorities must involve some analysis of whether the expenditure is part of a commitment made in the past (e.g. the staffing of a hospital built many years ago) or as expenditure which will require funding over future periods (e.g. the maintenance of a new operating theatre installed during the current year). Second, in order to analyse trends of expenditure over several years it is wise to separate out those items which represent the cost of maintaining existing services from the provision for new services, for which very large sums of money are required at the very start. If this distinction is not made, there is a danger that total expenditure patterns over a period of several years will not reflect the fact that expensive projects were started in some years and not in others. Taking an example over ten years, it can be seen from Figure 14 that a project was started in year 2 and another in year 6. Assuming for simplicity's sake that these two projects were new wings of an existing hospital and that the building was completed in one year, it can be seen that each of the new wings requires revenue expenditure in all subsequent years for running costs. If only the bottom line (total expenditure) was taken, this would give a distorted picture for analysis of increased costs over the period.

Third, it is necessary for purposes of comparison between NHS regions and also for comparison of expenditure on the NHS and other government spending departments to make such a distinction. Capital expenditure almost always involves large sums of money and, unless the distinction was made, public expenditure would be difficult to plan. Capital projects which were necessary for the adequate maintenance of existing assets (e.g. replacing worn-out equipment) might otherwise not get sufficient priority, bearing in mind the scarce resources available to the public sector. Fourth, in judging the timing of expenditure, current items represent a continuing financial commitment which cannot normally be significantly reduced. Capital commitments on the other hand can be brought forward or postponed depending on a government's overall economic strategy. In precise terms, this means that there is normally no possibility of deciding that hospital sheets should not be laundered or that nurses should not be paid, whereas the building of a new hospital can be delayed for one or two years if the government wishes to save money in the current year.

The rigid application of the distinction between capital and revenue expenditure has, in the past, been criticised for discouraging local managers from using their discretion to finance services in a flexible and economic way. It also used to be the rule that all unspent money should be returned at the end of the financial year, thus penalising those authorities who, through wise financial management, had been able to achieve economies. They found that their underspending could

Figure 14 *Capital and Current Expenditure*

YEARS	£ million — excluding inflation									
	1	2	3	4	5	6	7	8	9	10
Current expenditure: original hospital premises	5	5	5	5	5	5	5	5	5	5
Current expenditure: first new wing			1	1	1	1	1	1	1	1
Current expenditure: second new wing							1	1	1	1
TOTAL CURRENT EXPENDITURE	5	5	6	6	6	6	7	7	7	7
Capital expenditure: first new wing		5								
Capital expenditure: second new wing						5				
TOTAL CAPITAL EXPENDITURE		5				5				
TOTAL (CAPITAL & CURRENT EXPENDITURE)	5	10	6	6	6	11	7	7	7	7

result in a reduced financial allocation for the following year. However, these anomalies have recently been recognised and health authorities are now permitted to carry over underspendings of up to 1 per cent of their budgets into the following year and to transfer up to 1 per cent of revenue allocation for capital spending and up to 10 per cent of capital allocation for revenue. Capital spending is now defined as acquisition of land or premises, individual works schemes costing £15,000 or more, purchases of equipment costing £7,500 or more, pay and expenses of works department staff and all vehicles.[1]

In addition, however, the discipline of cash limits now operates in the NHS (and other public services). This means that the health authorities are notified of their capital and revenue allocations for the year, out of which they are obliged to meet all their commitments for that year. Any overspending they make is recovered from them by making a corresponding deduction from their allocation for the following year. The system of cash limits is different from income and expenditure accounting in that it does not allow for accounts outstanding or for stocks in hand. It was introduced to reduce problems with the government's cash-flow. One further discipline which was introduced in 1976 relates to the revenue consequences of capital schemes (RCCS). As Figure 14 shows, the consequence of making capital spending is to increase revenue spending in subsequent years (if the capital was spent in order to develop services). Previously this was acknowledged by adding the estimated amount of the increase to health authorities' allocations. This process has now ceased, so in order to finance the RCCS that health authorities incur, they have to use part of their ordinary revenue allocation, which does not contain any special extra amount apart from planned growth monies (if any) voted by parliament each year. The effect, because of cash limits, is to require the health authorities to make savings from other elements of their revenue expenditure.

In order to pay for the NHS and personal social services money is derived from three sources as shown in Figure 15: central and local government funds, the NHS element of National Insurance contributions and charges paid by users. Until the 1974 reorganisation community health services were paid for out of the local authority rates and Exchequer rate support grants, but they are now financed from the health authorities' allocations. However, personal social services and environmental health services continue to be financed through the local authorities.

The NHS contribution is an earmarked sum that was paid by employers and employees as part of their weekly National Insurance stamps. After April 1975 this contribution was derived mainly from the National Insurance payments which were collected through the PAYE system. Payments to the NHS by users of its services were not included in the original conception – which had aimed to secure a comprehensive system of health care, available free of charge on the basis of need alone. But from 1951, governments found that an accelerating rate of public expenditure in an unstable economic climate forced them to recoup some of the cost through charges to patients. These include payments for prescriptions, dentures, courses of dental treatment, spectacle lenses, surgical and medical appliances. However large numbers of patients were and have continued to be exempt, so that over 60 per cent of drug prescriptions are free, as are 48 per cent of dental treatments, and only 34 per cent of the cost of the General Ophthalmic service (not hospital) was, by 1977, recovered from patients. Payments for patients occupying beds in NHS hospitals for private treatment were instituted right at the beginning, and this income is now included as a part of the authorities' funds for revenue spending.[2]

Figure 15 *Sources of Finance: Health and Personal Social Services*

	£m(1984/5)	%
1 Central and local government exchequer Exchequer votes Rate support grant Local authority rates	12,796	83
2 National Insurance contributions	1,820	12
3 Charges paid by users	805	5
	15,421	100

How the Government Pays

The major source of income, from the Consolidated Fund, is not automatically administered from year to year, but only made available after an intricate process of negotiation within the central government machinery. Reference was made, in Chapter 2, to the relationship between the DHSS and the Treasury in connection with the development of policies. This relationship is at the heart of the way money is obtained for spending on the health service, and particularly concerns the public services divisions of the Treasury. These divisions are key elements of the Treasury, where all national government expenditure is supervised, through a series of consultations throughout the year with the spending departments, Treasury Ministers and the Cabinet. Each spring, all the spending departments (e.g. the DHSS, the Department of the Environment, the Department of Trade and Industry, the Ministry of Defence) submit preliminary returns to the Treasury. These are prepared in accordance with guidelines agreed by the Cabinet. They outline the revalued figures for the four years covered by the previous plan, with proposals for any new expenditure and for possible savings, together with figures for the new fifth year. They take account of a Cabinet discussion of the medium-term economic outlook and of their priorities, as well as of detailed economic assumptions provided by the Treasury. In proposing them, the departmental officials confer with their Ministers in order to work out their proposals for the continuation of existing policies and the development of new ones. This process is not always straightforward since there may well be disagreement about what current policy actually is. Then from March to May the officials of the departments have very detailed discussions with officials from the public services division in order to agree on statistical assumptions and their effect on the projected future cost of existing policies. In May the Principal Finance Officers from each spending department meet together with officials from the General Expenditure Division of the Treasury, and write a report which projects the future cost of all the national policies as they stand, and defines the areas where agreement has yet to be reached.

Their report is called the Public Expenditure Survey Committee (PESC) Report, and it is a key document on which the government's subsequent deliberations are based. The Principal Finance Officers, although officials of their own departments, need to foster the closest confidential relations with the Treasury in order that they may give their own department an accurate picture of the proposals that are likely to be successful with the Treasury, and those that will need persuasion to be acceptable. When they meet their opposite numbers to draw up the PESC report, they are in a position to assess the likely balance of demands for new spending between competing departments and they attempt to get as much as they reasonably can for their own departments, without antagonising the Treasury officials. The process depends very much at this stage on the trusting and cooperative nature of the relationships between these officials.

The next stage of the process involves the Treasury Ministers. They receive the PESC report (as does each of the departments) and, together with Treasury officials study the effect of its expenditure proposals in the light of their assessment of the economic climate and the government's strategy. They have to decide whether the proposals could actually be paid for with the sources that are likely to be available. The Chancellor of the Exchequer's view is presented to the Cabinet, and exceptionally he may find that increased spending will be possible in some areas, but more often he suggests that some cuts in the projections of individual departments will have to be made. The Cabinet argues over these points, and individual Ministers have to try to persuade their colleagues over the precedence of their claims for resources. Much may depend on whether the Prime Minister (who chairs Cabinet meetings) is in favour of certain policies rather than others. He or she will have already had confidential meetings with the Chancellor and the Secretary of the Cabinet, and his or her own mind may be made up before the Cabinet meets. Nevertheless, the discussions continue from June to November after which the Cabinet's decisions are embodied in the White Paper on Public Expenditure, which is published early the next year. It is subsequently debated for two days in the House of Commons, but this is now usually a formality and few if any amendments are made to it. The House's Select Committee on Expenditure (which succeeded the Select Committee on Estimates in 1970) chooses topics in the White Paper for study by each of its six sub-committees, and reports on its findings to the House of Commons. Although this represents a more critical look at policy decisions than the debate on the White Paper achieves, its influence on the proposals which are, after all, largely constructed by departmental officials, is relatively small, because the MPs do not always have the grasp of the broad issues and forward implications of decisions that the full-time officials can develop. This is, however, an area where MPs could exert more influence over future government policy, if they chose to play a more active part. The PESC plans are converted to up-to-date prices and set out in a form in which Parliament actually votes the money for the year ahead. At the same time, a cash limit is calculated incorporating projections of future inflation and representing the limit on the amount of extra money which the departments can expect on grounds of price increases.

Once Parliament has agreed to the allocations for each department, through the annual 'Votes', its involvement is temporarily ended. Later in the financial year that the vote covers, departments may, through their Ministers, come back for more money (subject to the overall cash limits); the Treasury puts forward requests for supplementary allocations after discussion with the departments, and Parliament agrees to allow the additional money. Parliament is subsequently involved in the scrutiny of departmental spending through the work of the Comptroller and Auditor General, and the investigations of its Public Accounts Committee – both of these were discussed in Chapter 2.

When the DHSS finally receives its allocation for the current year, it is able to pass money on to the Regions and Districts in accordance with their previously agreed budgets. Requests for new cash are made in the middle of the week for the five days of the next week. This amount is sufficient for the officers to write cheques in payments of goods and services. Some requests for money go straight to the DHSS and some go to the RHA, depending partly on how the Regional finance department is equipped – many have computers to handle the payroll, in which case all salaries and wages for Regional and District staff (i.e. the biggest single element of spending) may be paid through it.

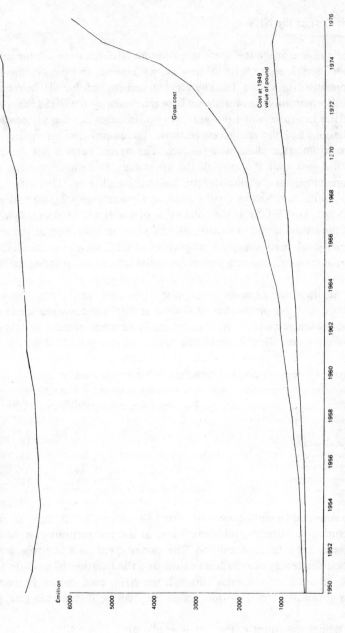

Figure 16 *The Cost of the National Health Service*

Cost as % of GNP

Gross cost

Cost at 1949 value of pound

£million

6000

5000

4000

3000

2000

1000

1950 1952 1954 1956 1958 1960 1962 1964 1966 1968 1970 1972 1974 1976

Source: OHE Compendium of Health Statistics, 1977

The Cost of the NHS

The amount of money being spent on the NHS has risen substantially. There are three ways of looking at the increase, and each of them is represented in Figure 16. The gross annual cost of the NHS produces the steepest curve, and it shows how much money the DHSS has spent on the health service from year to year. But this figure is affected by inflation, and the second curve shows the annual cost when the rise due to inflation alone is discounted. The second curve is not as steep as the first, but it shows all the same that the definite trend is for more money to be allocated to the DHSS each year. The last curve represents expenditure on the NHS as a percentage of gross national product (GNP). GNP is the total value of goods and services produced by the nation and is conventionally taken as an indication of the level of national resources. The proportion of GNP spend on the NHS is also increasing, but at a slower rate than the actual spending of the NHS.

All these trends make more sense when they are compared against others, and the proportion of GNP that different countries spend on their health services is one that can easily be made because its calculation is not complicated by currency exchange-rate considerations.

Figure 17 *Proportion of GNP Spent on Health Services*

	% GNP	Year
Sweden	9.8	1977
USA	9.4	1980
West Germany	9.2	1978
France	8.4	1979
Netherlands	8.2	1977
United Kingdom	5.6	1980

However, different countries' expenditure on health care is not recorded in strictly equivalent ways, so the comparisons have to be interpreted with some caution. The money spent does not necessarily buy a 'better' system of health care, and the question of whether the UK gets 'value for money' through the NHS, even though it spends proportionally less than other countries, will be discussed in Chapter 13.

Within the country, the resources allocated to the NHS can also be compared with other items of public expenditure. Some items are intrinsically more costly than others so any conclusions from the

Figure 18 *Analysis of Public Expenditure*

	£m cash (1984/5)
Social security	37,207
Defence	17,031
Health and personal social services	15,421
Education and science	13,052
Trade, industry, energy and employment	5,609
Law, order and protective services	4,901
Transport	4,372
Other environmental services	3,451
Housing	2,496
Overseas aid and other overseas services	2,283
Agriculture, fisheries, food and forestry	2,048
Nationalised industries external finance	1,881
Other programmes including Scotland, Wales and Northern Ireland	17,632
Adjustments	850
Total	126,353

Source: The Government's Expenditure Plans 1984/5–1986/7 (Cmnd. 9143-I)

comparison need to be carefully made. Figure 18 shows that for all items of public expenditure, the health and personal social services fall into third place, exceeded (in spending terms) by social security payments and defence. In 1984/5 all public expenditure amounted to £126,400m, of which the health and personal social services received 12.2 per cent. The total public expenditure amounted to 42 per cent of GDP for that year.

Looking more closely at the distribution of expenditure between the different elements of the health and personal social services, their relative positions as suggested by successive Public Expenditure White Papers is only gradually changing, even though the Personal Social Services have been given financial priority. This is because the hospitals' dominant position is so fixed that differential rates of expansion set out in the White Papers can only have a mild effect on the distribution of the total allocation from the DHSS. If a more substantial and radical change was required, the largest element of revenue expenditure for the hospitals − salaries and wages − would have to be switched to the preferred sector. As the discussion of capital and revenue expenditure at the beginning of the chapter indicated, the creation of new sources of revenue commitments through building new hospitals and expanding old ones has consequences for many years on. When William Beveridge proposed a comprehensive national health scheme in his 1944 report, he was convinced that its cost would stay at under £200 million per annum because the effects of its action on ill-health would steadily create a healthier population who had no further need for its services, so the scheme would not have to expand. His optimism was a serious miscalculation, since it is now apparent that a finite demand for health care does not exist. There is no guarantee that if 20 per cent or 50 per cent or even 100 per cent of funds allocated for public expenditure were given to the NHS, that the population would eventually cease to make more demands upon the services.

The Distribution of Resources

A breakdown of spending on the NHS (see Figure 19) shows that the hospitals started off with about 55 per cent of the total, which rose to over 65 per cent in the first 25 years of the NHS. Consequently the other sectors had to have a reduced share, so spending on general medical services fell in the same period from 10 per cent to about 6 per cent, and general dental services went from 8 per cent to 4 per cent, although there was an overall increase in the spending on family practitioner services. Any substantial alterations could only come through such drastic measures as the closure of many hospitals or the creation of a large fund to permit increased capital and revenue spending in the non-hospital sectors.

This chapter has not yet tackled the question of whether the NHS spends its money in the most effective way, and whether the reorganisation could have any influence in this respect. The 1972 White Paper on the reorganisation (1972) announced that, '. . . the allocations of available funds to health authorities will be designed progressively to reduce the disparities between the resources available to different regions, and to achieve standards and improvements in services with due regard to national, regional and area priorities'.[3]

The figures for staff working in the NHS are shown in Figure 20, and Figure 21 shows that hospital and community services take up nearly two thirds of the total. Pay is the largest part of total revenue spending – 55 per cent. It is also interesting to note that although total expenditure on the hospital sector accounts for over half the NHS budget, only 3 per cent of patients are cared for as inpatients each year. 81 per cent of patients are seen by general practitioners, and 16 per cent have outpatient treatment. Some of the regional inequalities that have resulted from the lack of planned distribution of financial and

Figure 19 *Analysis of Spending on Each Service*

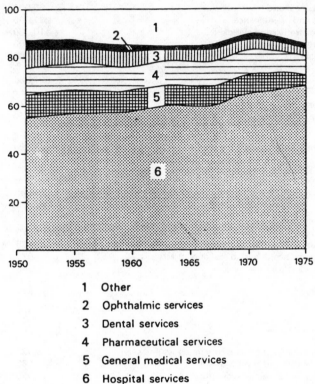

% NHS expenditure

1 Other
2 Ophthalmic services
3 Dental services
4 Pharmaceutical services
5 General medical services
6 Hospital services

Source: OHE Compendium of Health Statistics, 1977

manpower resources are shown in Figure 22. Solving the problems this has created does not simply require more and more money to be spent on the NHS. Available funds for most public services in the UK now fall short of demand because it is felt that the share of national income devoted to the public sector should not grow rapidly while the country's overall economic growth rate is so low.

Figure 20 *NHS Hospital and Community Staff*

	Numbers*
Medical and dental	40,000
Nursing and midwifery	397,000
Professional and technical	69,000
Works and maintenance	27,000
Administrative and clerical	110,000
Ambulance	18,000
Ancillary	166,000
Total	827,000

* Approximate totals, England, 1983
Source: The Government's Expenditure Plans 1984/5–1986/7 (Cmnd. 9143-II)

Figure 21 *Expenditure and Income: Health and Personal Social Services*

	£m cash (1984/5)
(a) *Spending: Services*	
Hospital and community health services	9,676
Family practitioner services	2,885
Central health and miscellaneous services	577
Personal social services	2,282
Total	15,421
(b) *Spending: Category*	
Pay	8,439
Other current expenditure on goods and services	6,025
Subsidies and current grants	85
Total current expenditure	14,550
Total capital expenditure	870
Total	15,421
(c) *Income from Charges**	
Hospital and community health services	75
Family practitioner services	344
Central health and miscellaneous services	9
Personal social services	377
Total	805

* England
Source: The Government's Expenditure Plans 1984/5–1986/7 (Cmnd. 9143-II)

Figure 22 *Regional Variations*

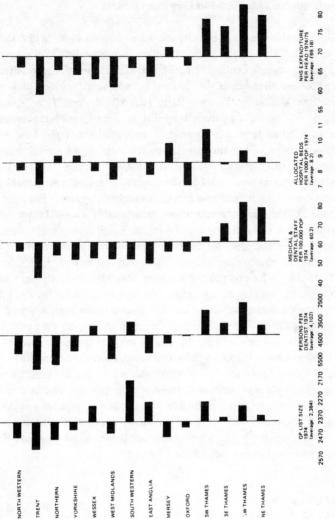

NORTH WESTERN
TRENT
NORTHERN
YORKSHIRE
WESSEX
WEST MIDLANDS
SOUTH WESTERN
EAST ANGLIA
MERSEY
OXFORD
SW THAMES
SE THAMES
W THAMES
NE THAMES

GP LIST SIZE
1974
(average: 2,384)

2570 2470 2370 2270 2170

PERSONS PER
DENTIST 1974
(average: 4,102)

5500 4500 3500 2500

MEDICAL &
DENTAL STAFF
PER 100,000 POP
1974
(average: 60.2)

40 50 60 70 80

ALLOCATED
HOSPITAL BEDS
PER 1000 POP 1974
(average: 8.2)

7 8 9 10 11

NHS EXPENDITURE
PER HEAD 1974/75
(average: £69.18)

55 60 65 70 75 80

Source: DHSS

The Resource Allocation Working Party (RAWP)

Achieving the equitable distribution of those funds the NHS does have depends on a workable policy for increasing spending in the deprived regions by correspondingly reducing the allocations to the better-off regions. The NHS began this process by adopting the principles of the Resource Allocation Working Party (RAWP) Report. This provided a scheme for calculating future 'target' allocations for each region according to a formula which takes into account the differential needs of various groups within the population for a range of hospital and community health services. Under the RAWP scheme the total NHS resources should be allocated to the regions in such a way that they can reach their 'targets' within a specified number of years.[4] The principles of the RAWP report could, over time, enable the NHS to provide services more fairly in relation to need, although successful implementation depends on, amongst other things, the health authorities' ability to construct appropriate strategic plans that can be realised within their cash limits.[5] The reorganised structure should be able to assist in this through its control mechanisms which are intended to coordinate the sum of individual local activity into a more logical whole. The medium of control is money and the method is based on the scrutiny of budgets and expenditure by each level over the next. The result is hopefully a more effective pattern of care, especially since the hospital and community services are now considered together as complementary and interdependent elements. However, in practice RAWP has been difficult to implement within Regions, because it requires a redistribution of resources. This cannot be done in some cases without making unacceptable cuts in the level of service. It seems unlikely that RAWP targets will be reached before the 1990s.

Joint Financing

Lack of resources in local authority social services departments has sometimes meant that patients have remained in hospital when they would have done better in the community. Cooperation between health and social services authorities could provide more appropriate care. However there were statutory obstacles to achieving this in that health authorities could not transfer resources to local authorities. So in 1976 a new arrangement was brought in allowing health authorities to fund developments in social services departments on the understanding that the cost would gradually be transferred. The Health Services Act 1980 Section 4 confirmed the new arrangements. Area Health Authorities being usually conterminous with county councils were able to develop the joint projects and good progress was made. However in the early 1980s increasing financial pressure on local authorities meant that they were less able to take on long-term commitments. Nevertheless a survey published in 1983[6] showed considerable support for joint financing as an effective way of planning and providing services together, despite the recognition that in many places the money had mostly been used to cushion local authority cuts. Government commitment remained and in 1982 the rules were altered to allow a much longer pay-back period.

Budgetary Control

The financial control system works in parallel with the planning cycle, and focuses on capital and revenue expenditure. It is exercised through the injunction that each level of authority monitors the planned and actual spending of the one below it. In practice this means that the DHSS sets down guidelines for the Regions to observe, and keeps an eye on them to see that this happens. Similarly, the Regions watch the way that the Districts keep within the limits they have set them, and the Districts watch the managers of Units and departments. Obviously, the more detail each level builds in to its guidelines for the one below it, the less freedom the lower one will have for variations, so the official view is that the degree of detail should be '. . . kept to the minimum necessary to preserve accountability'.[7]

Budgets serve three main functions in commercial organisations — planning, controlling and costing. In the NHS these functions traditionally had low priority, but with the reorganisation there are now closer parallels between commercial organisations and the operation of the NHS. The role that budgets play in the planning cycle has already been discussed; it is clear that without making estimates of future spending and assessing their relative importance in this systematic way, it would be extremely difficult to build a realistic model of the way the NHS should develop, or to influence planning decisions so that this is facilitated. Since budgeting and planning were generally so poorly used in the pre-1974 NHS, they failed to provide the comprehensive and efficient scheme of care that was originally envisaged. The planning cycle itself is a model that was unlikely to be put into practice as precisely as its designers would have liked. Two factors, the ever-rising bill for public expenditure to be met by a government with a huge balance of payments deficit, and the relative newness of many NHS staff to the discipline of forward planning, meant that the cycle had to start in difficult 'operating conditions' that were not guaranteed to improve in the near future. It does however represent the DHSS's commitment to the view that unless a more systematic control was exercised over the NHS, they would not be able to have confidence in its future.

Control is the second function of budgets mentioned above, and it means that by comparing the use of his allocated resources regularly during the year with his budget, a manager (e.g. of a service or a department) has a reliable way of assessing his work, and of altering certain elements in the light of this. The budget is not simply about how fast the allocated money is being spent, since it can provide details of such factors as the productivity of staff, the efficiency of machines, and the changing cost of supplies. In commercial organisations the budget also serves as a control against total overspending, but in the NHS, although this is true, unanticipated spending caused by factors outside the manager's control, e.g. increased salaries and wages bills resulting from nationally negotiated pay awards, or increased spending on raw materials caused by rising prices in an inflationary situation, is to some extent compensated for by supplementary allocations on top of the cash limit which are negotiated by the DHSS. It was shown earlier that the Treasury builds into its plans for public expenditure certain amounts which are provided to departments when this sort of overspending is unavoidably incurred.

The budget also indicates the amount of money to be spent on individual items (as well as the total amount) and these sums can be analysed to show the costing of the service that they produce. In other words, the value of resources used up in providing different types of service can be identified from information contained in the budget. This use of costing in a commercial organisation, even if it is a service enterprise (as opposed to a manufacturing one) is straightforward to apply, and essential for the calculation of profit margins. The NHS, on the other hand, has no concept of profit, nor does it have a reliable definition of its objectives against which performance can be assessed. The useful information contained in the budgets has not, as a consequence, been fully exploited, and many ineffective and wasteful practices (both clinical and administrative) have persisted. However, this situation has not gone unnoticed and papers and reports have been appearing since the 1960s confirming the problems of the costing system and suggesting various reforms. In a sense, the whole 1974 reorganisation was a reaction to the problem since its stated objectives were to unify the administration of health care in the interests of achieving a better quality of service from the existing expenditure. The attitudes of doctors are relevant here because by maintaining the medical profession's freedom to direct the use of such a large part of the available resources without stringent controls, the task of management to obtain better value for money in the NHS is made harder. Doctors are allowed to treat individual patients as they think best, yet DMTs and health authorities have to have policies which will control doctors' activities without interfering in them.

Increasingly attempts are being made to introduce more cost awareness into the NHS. Whilst concepts from market economics may be inappropriate to a service based more on needs than on demands, it cannot be denied that there is room for a more rigorous approach to the efficient use of resources. Clinical budgeting is an attempt to make those who treat patients fully aware of the financial consequences of their actions. It is distinct from costing, which provides common standards of comparison, so that, for instance, the cost of catering in one hospital can be compared with that in another. But there are few incentives (other than for administrators), to take action on the results of these comparisons. Another shortcoming is that costing is a retrospective exercise which may be dismissed because present circumstances have changed.

On the other hand, clinical budgeting looks forward and cannot take place without the involvement of clinicians. By this process doctors have to become involved in the setting up of budgets. They are thus made more conscious of the cost of the services they are giving to patients. Once the budget is set, regular reviews of expenditure are conducted by the doctor and his team. If savings are made they are potentially available to be redistributed by the budget holder. This may create a strong incentive to underspend. However, clinical budgeting is more expensive to run and because hospital services depend on complicated inter-dependencies between different departments and teams, it is not easy to isolate budgets under one budget holder. For instance, should nurses be seen as part of a medical specialty or as part of the overall nursing service? In the former case the medical budget holder, the doctor, would have the power to reduce the number of nurses on his ward and re-deploy the savings. But this would be unacceptable to a chief nurse responsible not only for the deployment of nurses throughout the whole hospital, but also for maintaining professional standards.

Despite these difficulties, clinical budgeting has been tried in several hospitals, starting with the Westminster Hospital in 1973/74, and it has proved to have considerable potential for better management of patient care.[8] Inherent in this method is a more explicit management structure with accountable budget holders.

Value for Money?

With regard to the objectives of the NHS, the kind of statements that are generally acceptable refer to obtaining the maximum benefit from the resources that are used, or maximising the health of the community for a given expenditure. But since there is no way of measuring health or of recognising maximum benefits, the choice between alternative types of care becomes very arbitrary. The trend is towards finding some way of measuring outputs of the NHS which will be useful indicators for management decisions, even if they are not absolutely unbiased definitions. Certain output statistics have been recorded for the hospital service since 1948. From the accounts, departments' spending is costed in relation to inpatients and day patients in each hospital. This provides figures for the unit costs of departments and for the average costs per inpatient week, and the average cost per 100 outpatient attendances. Inpatients and outpatients are divided according to clinical specialty, and total outpatient attendances and inpatient admissions are counted under these headings. The data that result from these analyses, although of some use to the hospitals concerned, are unreliable as a record of national activity since there are many sources of error built into them. In 1965 a new system, called Hospital Activity Analysis (HAA) was introduced; for each inpatient date of birth, sex, marital status, area of residence, length of stay, hospital, consultant and specialty are recorded. This gives information about rates of discharges and deaths and differential lengths of stay between specialties and hospitals and consultants, that can be used for comparisons between hospitals and regions. Maternity and mental illness admissions are not always recorded in this scheme, but if all admissions were included and the system could link individual records (to allow for more than one admission per person) HAA would be able to compare performance in different areas more reliably, and would also show details of the way patients are referred for inpatient care, both within and between areas.

Without accurate information of this kind, NHS planners cannot make proper decisions about adjustments to services, since they cannot be fully aware of the current situation. HAA is also used to provide information for the Hospital Inpatient Enquiry (HIPE); this is a 10 per cent sample of the discharges recorded through HAA returns, and it is published annually. As far as general practice is concerned, routine information is not collected but there are special studies done from time to time.[9] These assessments of workload do not match in strength the analyses of NHS costs, so by relating the two to each other, information of consistent reliability cannot be ensured. Only by comparing measures of performance within one unit or institution can managers develop sound yardsticks that will guide them in working towards their objectives.

Four successive systems of cost accounting have been introduced in the NHS, the most recent being in 1973. This latest one does permit some functional outputs to be assessed and compared according to specialty, but as with its predecessors, it gives no way of judging how well resources are being used, and this is the item that is so urgently needed. Advances in techniques of treatment and the invention of new drugs contribute to the quality of care as do the screening programmes, but the problem is in deciding whether these are more desirable outputs, i.e. whether they are preferentially increasing the health of the population. One economic technique that was regarded in the 1960s as the new breakthrough in evaluating alternative choices of public expenditure policy is 'cost-benefit analysis'. Cost-benefit analysis is a way of analysing intended spending of public money to enable the maximum social advantage to be obtained.

The technique has been applied to a range of other projects, including forms of treatment used in the NHS. One example is the introduction of cervical smears in the hope of detecting cancer of the cervix in its early stages and treating it before it becomes intractable. About 4,000 women in Britain die from this disease each year and a nationwide screening service was available costing about £3 million each year. However, the number of lives, if any, that the screening saves is unknown. The assumptions on which it is based (e.g. that the early 'pre-cancerous' stage always progresses to clinical cancer, and that the 'pre-cancerous' stage lasts long enough to be detected by the smear programme) have still to be proved. The cost of treating 'pre-cancerous' cases in hospital, combined with the greater demand for smears from women in the higher social classes mean that it is almost impossible to evaluate the results of the screening programme. The decision to introduce it was taken in response to quite widespread public demand rather than on any clear economic assessment of the implications of the programme. Until 1982 this service was organised centrally by the DHSS from an office in Southport, Lancs. In 1982 the national service was wound up by the government in favour of local arrangements, which might be more sensitive to screening women particularly at risk. Although it cannot be demonstrated that more lives are being saved, the fact that a number of women *feel* better protected from death by cancer of the cervix is undeniably a benefit. This example shows that there is no absolute way of calculating whether a given proposal is worth what it will cost. So, although cost-benefit analysis does not provide unequivocal guidance for health service planning decisions, it does clarify the areas where value judgements have inevitably to be made. As one official from the DHSS has said, ' . . . if decisions do go against the logic of economic argument, it seems to me to be still right that the economic costs of making the decision should be established'.[10]

This points to the conclusion that medical care, at this stage in its history, provides tangible benefits in terms of the quality of health that individuals and their families can enjoy, but these are not necessarily convertible into quantifiable economic benefits that can justify consistently increasing public expenditure on the NHS. Consequently, some critics have proposed an alternative system of finance for the health service, in which the user pays for the cost of his treatment. The arguments are based on the view that the consumption of medical care is excessive when consumers do not pay directly for what they receive. Given that some form of rationing does exist, individual users should make the decisions about what to consume on the basis of price, instead of departmental officials doing this through their administrative decisions. Furthermore, it is said that a better standard of care would develop if treatment was available in a free market, because unnecessary 'frivolous' demand would be eliminated, true priorities for health expenditure would become clear and doctors and hospitals would raise the quality of their services in order to maintain their incomes. This point needs further examination with particular reference to the private sector of health care.

In a free market, supply is not controlled by government but instead responds to the demands of its users. In health care terms for this system to apply several assumptions have to be made. First, all market users must have equal opportunities to make demands on health care services. This is plainly not the case and was one of the fundamental reasons the NHS was set up in the first place; the disadvantaged needed help and protection. Secondly, a market is not really free if it is bound by any form of monopoly. In health care many groups of professionals operate monopolies, pre-eminently the doctors. So users of the NHS have little choice but to accept the doctor and his control of the resources. Thirdly, a user of a health care system has little basis on which to judge whether the quality of what he is getting is better or worse than what he might have had. Quality in health care is difficult to assess except by retrospective judgements which conclude that people are in some sense 'better-off' than they were before they became users of the service.

Another factor associated with free markets is that competition between suppliers reduces prices to users and drives the inefficient suppliers out of business. Although parts of the NHS could do more to reduce waste and to be more sensitive to patient demand, there is no question of the services 'going out of business' as long as existing legislation prevails. This places on the government the duty to provide comprehensive services for the treatment of disease and the prevention of ill-health. Private hospitals are not bound by this legal duty.

Even though the market economy model is inappropriate for the provision of health care in Britain, it is important to look further at alternative methods of funding. The most often discussed is the suggestion that a charge should be made to every patient who in turn would be obliged to be insured for health care costs. The Royal Commission pointed out[11] that there were many types of insurance schemes but all failed in the end to provide satisfactory protection for those poor patients at high risk from ill-health for whom the NHS already expends over 60 per cent of its funds. Insurance schemes are more suitable for meeting short-term needs for care than for providing preventive and long-term protection. The experience of other countries suggests that insurance funding would undoubtedly lead to higher administrative costs.

In addition, the NHS could supplement the resources it gets from central government by some degree of local funding either through local taxation or by using money from charities and voluntary bodies, or that collected by lotteries. Even if the sums available were significant (which must be doubted), there would be a serious distorting effect on equity within a national service. Nevertheless, the growth of the private sector alongside the NHS has been noticeable. Partly this has been provoked by increasing consumer dissatisfaction with particular aspects of the NHS (e.g. waiting lists, impersonal care), but it is also because of the political ideology of the government since 1979 which has been supportive to the growth of the private health care business.

Governments and Private Health Care

In August 1975 the DHSS published a consultative document called *The Separation of Private Practice from National Health Service Hospitals* which set out proposals to reduce the number of pay beds in NHS hospitals and to control developments in alternative private practice, in line with the government's stated commitment to this policy. The proposals met with fierce opposition in a number of quarters, and some hospital doctors were particularly hostile to them. The issue of private practice had been an element in the consultants' dispute with the government in 1974–75. Nevertheless, the *Health Services Bill* was published in April 1976 taking some of the objections into account, and after Parliamentary debate the *Health Services Act* received Royal Assent on 22 November 1976. It enabled the Secretary of State to promote the separation of facilities available for private practice from NHS premises, while protecting consultants' right to engage in private practice. 1,000 of the 4,444 private beds in NHS hospitals were withdrawn by May 1977 and made available, wherever possible, for the use of NHS patients. The Act created the Health Services Board which had to recommend which 1,000 beds should go within the first six months and had to propose further withdrawals of private beds and private outpatient facilities from NHS hospitals, taking into account representations from any interested parties. In addition, the Board had to make proposals within the first six months for the introduction of common waiting lists for private and NHS patients. It also had to control the authorisation of private hospitals and nursing homes so that the interests of the NHS and its patients would not be disadvantaged. The Board was disbanded by the *Health Services Act 1980*.

From the patient's point of view, private health care ensures that treatment will be obtained from a chosen consultant, a private single room will be available in hospital, the date of an outpatient consultation can be fixed quickly, the date of admission can be planned with a significantly shorter wait than would be involved for an NHS bed, and the sheer amount of attention from the private doctor is likely to be far greater than in an NHS setting. But the choice of private care is costly in that the patient has to pay for the hospital's 'hotel' services (which currently involve several hundred pounds per week) together with the fees of the doctor, anaesthetist, and other special staff, and costs of any tests, dressings and drugs. Insurance to cover some of this expenditure is available, and a survey carried out for the DHSS in 1974[12] showed that over 2¼ million people were covered by insurance schemes, although over 90 per cent of them were registered with NHS general practitioners. The great majority of people are covered through group subscriptions arranged by their employers. The three major private medical insurance agencies are BUPA (the British United Provident Association founded in 1947), the Western Provident Association (based in Bristol) and the London Association for Hospital Services (which operates the scheme called Private Patients Plan).

However, private health care is not comprehensively available in parallel with the NHS. Bevan's negotiations with the medical profession in 1946 enshrined in the National Health Service Act the right of GPs and consultants to take paying patients in addition to their NHS work. In practice over 90 per cent of GPs work totally within the NHS or have very few private patients whereas about half of all NHS consultants hold part-time contracts and undertake private work as well. Since 1948 hospitals had been permitted a quota of pay beds and in 1976 the total was 4,444 of which over 25 per cent were in London: Wales, Scotland and some regions of England had less than 100 each. This number declined rapidly so that by 1982 there were only 2,929. However, during that time there had been considerable expansion of private hospital beds. Opportunities for private practice are greater in some specialties than in others. Most geriatricians, venereologists and radiologists for example hold full-time contracts, while few ophthalmologists, ear nose and throat specialists or gynaecologists do. So the private sector offers most benefits to patients who want surgical care, particularly for those procedures (e.g. hip replacements, repair of hernia and varicose veins) where NHS waiting lists are long. But for longer-term hospital care the option barely exists because people with psychiatric disorders or mental handicap, who together constitute the largest group of hospital inpatients, could hardly afford to pay for months or years of care in private hospitals. There is room for some further growth in the private sector, but it cannot currently offer an alternative on a scale comparable to the NHS for general practitioner and non-acute hospital services to the majority of the population if it is to be run economically.

In conclusion, it must be emphasised that whatever the political views regarding private practice, it still only involves some 2 per cent of patients. This being so, the financial consequences of offloading some patients to private care outside the NHS, or recovering charges from private patients being treated in NHS hospitals, are small compared with the overall task of financing the NHS itself. The issue is therefore best understood in political terms. Supporters and critics of private practice are really arguing about their opinions of the State's duty to intervene where a free market is absent, and about the nature of these interventions.

Notes

1. Department of Health and Social Security. *Health Services Development: Cash Limits and the Health Capital Programme: Revised Definition of Capital Spending.* Health Circular HC(77)6, DHSS, London, March 1977. Revised from 1 April 1981. Circular FM 2/81 Appendix 4.

2. Not returned to the hospital are the reductions in social security benefit to these patients receiving benefit who are in hospital for a long time. After eight weeks the benefit is reduced by 40 per cent (20 per cent if these are dependents) and after a year to 20 per cent. Another source of income is the Road Traffic Act charges whereby a notional sum is charged to an accident victim's insurer.

3. *National Health Service Reorganisation: England*, HMSO, London 1972 (Cmnd. 5055), p. 40 para. 160.

4. RAWP was set up by the DHSS in 1975. It produced an Interim Report later that year and a further report in Autumn 1976 called *Sharing Resources for Health in England* (HMSO). The 1976 report contained the formula for redistributing both capital and revenue resources, and it also included a basis for calculating the extra allocations for clinical teaching and research. The report stressed that RHAs should in turn adopt the overall principles when calculating their allocations to the Areas and Districts, so that relative need for health services within the populations concerned was kept as the guiding theme.

5. The detail of the RAWP formula has however met with some criticism that it fails to measure 'need' for health services accurately enough, particularly if it is to be used exactly as set out in the report for calculating Area and District allocations. In addition, distribution of GP services (the responsibility of the Medical Practices Committee) is not covered by RAWP or the planning system, although it is known to be a key to the level of use of hospital and community resources. Until the MPC becomes more effective or GPs are brought into the planning system, the assumptions of the RAWP formula may be inadequate, even though they are currently the best available. For a critical review of RAWP see *Allocating Health Resources*, Royal Commission on the National Health Service Research Paper No. 3, HMSO, 1978.

6. National Association of Health Authorities and Centre for Research in Social Policy, Loughborough University. *Joint Planning in Perspective 1976-1982*, NAHA, Birmingham, 1983.

7. Department of Health and Social Security. *Management Arrangements for the Reorganised National Health Service*, HMSO, London, 1972, p. 57. para. 3.42a.

8. For a review of clinical budgeting experiments see: *British Medical Journal*, vol. 286, pp. 575–578.

9. For instance Ritchie, Jacoby and Bone. *Access to Primary Health Care*, HMSO, London, 1981.

10. H.C. Salter in: M.M. Hauser (ed.), *The Economics of Medical Care,* Allen and Unwin, London, 1972.

11. *Royal Commission on the National Health Service,* pp. 335–344, HMSO, London, 1979 (Cmnd. 7615).

12. Lee Donaldson Associates, *UK Private Medical Care; Provident Schemes Statistics,* Report to the DHSS, Lee Donaldson Associates, London, 1980.

PLANNING SERVICES FOR PATIENTS

The NHS Act 1946 in its opening statement made it clear that the new health service would be for everyone; it was not just a service for the sick. Has this grand intention been satisfied? This chapter looks at how services for various groups of patients and clients have developed. First, there is a historical account of the rise of planning within the NHS and then a description of the planning process since 1974. The chapter then reviews each care group referring to those events, surveys and reports which have had the most significant effect on policy.

Planning in the NHS 1948-74

Chapter 1 showed that the demand for a national health service emerged from the recognition that health care was ill-coordinated and under-provided. Substantial demands had been made during the Second World War which had not been adequately met. The creation of the NHS in 1948 was therefore expected to pave the way to better planned service for the future. The 1945 Labour government wanted to introduce the NHS as a key part of its overall design of the new welfare state. But any party forming a government then would have had to have proposals to deal with health care needs. Early on in the NHS rising expenditure became a major problem and in 1953 the Guillebaud Committee was set up to examine the financing of the service. Their report in 1956[1] exonerated the NHS from the accusation of wasteful use of resources. The Conservative government was forced, therefore, to plan for the best use of NHS resources in a more systematic manner.

One result of this was the publication in 1962 of *A Hospital Plan for England and Wales* (the 1962 Plan),[2] which might be said to be the first major demonstration of a concern for planning in the NHS, a concern which has gradually become an unavoidable discipline and lies behind the main reasons for both the 1974 and 1982 reorganisations.

The 1962 Plan acknowledged that capital expenditure was increasing from £8.7 million in 1949/50 to over £31 million in 1962/63. What was lacking was a sense of overall purpose; the capital schemes were largely *ad hoc* solutions to local problems. 'The moment has therefore come to take a comprehensive view of the hospital service as it is today and to draw the outlines of the service which we mean to create.'[3]

The 1962 Plan reviewed the existing provision of beds, suggesting norms for each major care group and integrated these in terms of specific proposals for each Region and within each Region for each hospital management committee. It needs to be emphasised that the 1962 Plan was about hospitals and about beds. It briefly acknowledged care in the community (a term to emerge almost as a slogan some 20 years later) and accepted that the development of hospital services must be complementary to developments in preventive and domiciliary care. Local health authorities were asked to review their services in conjunction with hospital authorities, but no consultative machinery was suggested and the overriding impression given by the 1962 Plan is that it was only really interested in hospital development. Not that this concern was ill directed. It has already been said in Chapter 1 that the state of the hospitals was unenviable. Over 45 per cent of them were built before 1891 and some 21 per cent before 1861. Many of this group were old workhouses now often used for geriatric patients. These buildings had mostly been constructed following the 1834 Poor Law Amendment Act. Emergency medical service (EMS) hospitals built at the beginning of the war were flexible because of their hutted single storey design. Due to the change in illness patterns, the time had come to re-use some of the other hospitals. Infectious diseases hospitals and sanitoria could quite easily be adapted for most uses, although they were often remotely situated. The 1962 Plan envisaged a gradual reorganisation of hospitals in order to build up a central district general hospital and reduce the number of small and outlying hospitals. A yearly review of progress was intended to assess changes of circumstance and the availability of capital resources. The 1962 Plan was relatively well received at the time, except that then as now, some of the proposed hospital closures raised public opposition. The process of centralisation and the 'bigger-is-better' movement was, however, in tune with the 1960s spirit of optimism and expansion and in this respect the 1962 Plan was well timed.

The 1962 Plan review of 1966[4] curbed some of the initial optimism and modified the original plans, but the basic philosophy was endorsed by the Bonham Carter Report published in 1969[5] which was devoted to describing the functions of the district general hospital. The logic of this report would have meant that some district general hospitals would have been very large indeed, possibly up to 1500 beds. As the number of hospitals with over 1,000 beds in England and Wales was very few this proposal did not find much support. But by failing to resolve the question of the optimum size of a district general hospital, many towns still have two such hospitals which creates waste due to the duplication of facilities.

No doubt an alarm at the high cost of the new district general hospital buildings and the increased revenue needed to run them led to a change of direction in 1975, with the publication of the DHSS paper on the development of community hospitals.[6] The 1962 Plan had concentrated on the district general hospital and the gradual closure of smaller hospitals. This proved to be unwise, because local opposition to closing down hospitals which had often been founded through local subscriptions proved to be powerful. In addition, such hospitals turned out to be cheaper to run than district general hospitals so savings could be made if not all patients were sent to the more expensive central district general hospital. The DHSS's criteria for admitting patients to community hospitals were that such patients needed medical and nursing care which could not normally be provided at home, but did not need the full range of district general hospital facilities. Secondly, it was seen as more humane to keep people as near to their own homes as possible, and in this respect the community hospital was particularly attractive for elderly patients whose visitors might also be elderly and less able to travel to a district general hospital miles away. The community hospital idea was not developed systematically during the 1970s partly because of the simultaneous upheavals facing the service, including reorganisation, and because of the substantial emphasis on better services for such care categories as the mentally handicapped and the mentally ill. Nevertheless the idea that there should be a balanced relationship between the district general hospital and local hospitals staffed by GPs is still topical and likely to remain a live issue for the next few years, given the renewed concern with the escalating costs of district general hospitals and the determination of local people to keep their local facilities.

The 1962 Plan and subsequent developments demonstrate the increasing concern in the NHS to plan in a systematic manner. Throughout the 1960s it was becoming apparent that such planning could not take place in a vacuum. Most people never go near a hospital, but still have a need of the health service. Attention needed to be given to improving hospital facilities and reviewing the needs of groups of patients on a wider basis, and to do this required cooperation with other branches of the NHS, particularly local health authorities. The original compromises made in 1946 had resulted in an NHS with three separately administered segments: the hospital service, family doctors and local health authorities. This division was proving an impediment to planning a better service. The Ministry of Health had published a local authority planning document in 1963 entitled *Health and Welfare – the Development of Community Care*,[7] but it was much less directive than the 1962 Plan, recognising that local authorities were more autonomous than Regional Hospital Boards. The 1974 reorganisation, therefore, was fuelled by the lack of systematic planning. Hospital management committees were happy enough running the hospitals on a day-to-day basis; their sense of what was needed in the future was poorly defined. For most administrators, plans were still a matter of bricks and mortar. The 1974 reorganisation changed this by suggesting there should be two types of administrator: one concerned with operational management (mostly found in the Districts) and another concerned with planning (mostly found at the Areas). Because this broad classification was too crude and simplistic it could not be worked in practice and was one of the reasons for the demise of Areas in 1982.

Given the means to plan, the DHSS made determined efforts to provide advice on planning procedures and policies. First the policies. *Priorities for Health and Personal Social Services in England* (Priorities document) was published in 1976.[8] The aim of this document was to make the priorities of the government more explicit whilst acknowledging the ever-present constraints, and to state that planning was a 'co-operative enterprise' involving the various tiers of the DHSS and NHS as well as local authorities and voluntary bodies. Only through this form of extended discussion could choices be made. Barbara Castle, the then Secretary of State emphasised that 'choice is never easy, but choose we must'.[9] The assumption behind this document was that if authorities were given the facts, they would decide upon priorities more readily. Studies of policy implementation suggest that this simple model of rational planning is out of touch with reality. *The Way Forward* 1977,[10] seemed to acknowledge that the comprehensiveness and detail of the Priorities document might not ensure its eventual success. *The Way Forward* was less specific about rates of increase in services and vaguer about time scales, whilst encouraging a continuing debate on priorities. Nevertheless, a general enthusiasm for planning remained and by this time AHAs were well into the process of providing guidelines for their Districts, collating District Plans and developing fruitful relationships with local authorities, particularly social services departments.

One way to encourage authorities to plan, was to change the rules for allocating resources to them. The adoption of the *Resources Allocation*

Working Party report (RAWP)[11] in 1976 required Regions to think much more carefully about what they were doing with their money. Those Regions likely to gain under RAWP clearly were encouraged, but the losers, particularly the London Regions, also had to examine their services with more care if the planned reductions were not to have a devastating effect.

Joint financing was first introduced in 1976[12] and provided earmarked money for schemes jointly agreed between health and social services departments. In May of the next year a further DHSS circular outlined in some detail the arrangements for joint financing of both capital and revenue schemes.[13] This initiative made a substantial difference to relationships between health authorities and local government. No longer did cooperation rely almost entirely on good faith as there was now money to be had and money which was restricted to particular use (the detailed arrangements were described in Chapter 6). Some initial difficulties were found with joint financing and not all authorities made use of the funds available. In 1979 and 1983 further amendments were made to overcome some of their problems, particularly by extending the period during which schemes could be financed from this special allocation.

Another policy initiative of the 1970s was the publication *Prevention and Health: Everybody's Business* in 1976.[14] Ignoring the terms of the 1946 NHS Act, health prevention had had little priority in explicit plans. This was despite the considerable success in improving the health of the nation. As the document pointed out, the death rate from tuberculosis and the other main infectious diseases had been substantially reduced. But these successes unmasked other health problems which needed to be tackled and the document called for discussion on the remaining and emerging problem areas. Although promoting good health was argued to be a cost effective activity, health authorities have been relatively slow to produce specific plans aimed at health promotion.

The history of health service planning during the last decade is the story of optimistic intentions later modified by caution. The Priorities document – remarkable for its detailed plans – was trimmed a year later by *The Way Forward*. Similarly, a note of caution was struck by the consultation paper issued in May 1980 by the Minister for Health, Dr Vaughan, entitled *Future Pattern of Hospital Provision in England*.[15] The paper put the brake on building district general hospitals. The Minister said this was necessary because of their escalating cost. During the 1970s attempts had been made to standardise the design of such hospitals with three different systems entitled Best Buy, Harness and Nucleus. It was hoped that standardisation would cut the design cost, and in the case of Harness and Nucleus, phased construction of hospitals could be implemented. Costly monoliths such as the Royal Liverpool Hospital at over £50 million had frightened the DHSS and health authorities alike. The paper proposed that district general hospitals should not normally exceed 600 beds and that smaller hospitals should be retained wherever 'sensible and practicable'.

There were two other important contributions to priority-setting: *Care in Action*[16] and *Care in the Community*,[17] both published in 1981. *Care in Action*, although published before the 1982 reorganisation, was addressed to the chairmen and the members of the new District health authorities. The pamphlet, described as a handbook of policies and priorities, aimed to help the new DHAs to take local initiatives, make local decisions and shoulder local responsibility. Local decision making was a general theme of the 1982 reorganisation and a reaction against the results of the top heavy 1974 formula. A separate (and shorter) preface was addressed to chairmen and members of social services committees emphasising the responsibility of health authorities to collaborate with social services committees and departments. *Care in Action* is different from the 1976 Priorities document in its emphasis on the range of options for health provision. Considerable importance is given to the potential contribution from the voluntary and private sectors. This theme of partnership was to be developed more strongly in later documents. *Care in Action* also emphasised the need for greater efficiency so that more patients could be seen for the same financial outlay. Community care was not only an alternative but a cheaper alternative to institutional care. *Care in the Community* had made this point strongly by saying that most people needing long-term care would prefer to remain at home as long as possible. This proposal was well supported by current opinion but was also fuelled by the less altruistic view that it would be cheaper to avoid the capital costs and a substantial proportion of the revenue costs of running these buildings. The voluntary organisations were seen as being able to play an important part in contributing to the support of the community. In 1983 the circular confirming the principles of *Care in the Community* allowed health authorities to extend the joint financing arrangements to voluntary bodies as well as social services departments. The circular went further by recommending that hospital buildings could be transferred to local authorities in order to accelerate the discharge of people from health authority administered institutional care. These two DHSS initiatives seemed to ignore the crucial message of the *Working Group on Inequalities in Health* 1980 (Black report),[18] which called for a frank recognition of the links between standards of health care and social class. It declared the pressing need for significant targeted funds over many years to really make good some of the greatest deprivation.

Following the 1982 reorganisation, planning took a new turn. The comprehensive overview of the service relying on norms for each care group had proved to be inflationary, encouraging an over-provision of facilities and manpower, which had proved increasingly embarrassing to the government. Looking back over the Priorities document and *Care in Action* and other advice of the middle and late 1970s, *everything* had become a priority. Realism now demanded less idealistic plans, particularly as the national economy had not improved at the expected rate.

There was increasing emphasis on efficiency, doing the same for less or doing more for the same; on partnership, getting voluntary bodies or the private sector to contribute to health care; and, with the report of the *NHS Management Inquiry* (Griffiths report),[19] on making decisions more quickly and ensuring that they were implemented. If the 1974 reorganisation of the NHS was the heyday of planning, the 1982 reorganisation seems set to be the period of concern with performance.

The Planning Process

The 1974 reorganisation created the first serious attempt to plan the health services in a systematic and comprehensive manner on a multi-disciplinary basis. Prior to this, most disciplines did not bother to plan rationally, or if they did, failed to take all interests into account. Health Care Planning Teams (HCPTs) were set up in 1974 to draw together professionals concerned with particular groups of clients or patients. The idea was that each team should examine the existing level of service and make recommendations to the DMT for improvements. The teams were formally approved by the AHA, but in practice membership and scope were decided and arranged by DMTs to whom HCPTs reported. Later HCPTs changed their title to District Planning Teams (DPTs) but their function remained the same.

The 1974 reorganisation also created Joint Consultative Committees (JCCs) within each Area made up of members of county councils and health authorities. These committees were serviced by the Area Team of Officers. Due to the time spent implementing reorganisation, these planning teams were slow to start work. In March 1975 the DHSS published a comprehensive handbook called *Guide to Planning in the National Health Service*,[20] which set out the detailed tasks to be performed at each level in the structure and explained the concept of both annual and strategic planning. The Guide was implemented in 1976 by a publication called the *NHS Planning System*.[21] So from a situation where little systematic planning was undertaken, especially at local level, an elaborate infrastructure had been established. This in its turn was to be officially criticised just five years later by *Patients First* for being too cumbersome. The *NHS Planning System* document endorsed the original 1972 proposals for an annual planning cycle which, modelled on the PESC system, prepared and processed plans at certain times of the year, allowing District plans for instance to arrive at the Region in time (it was thought) to influence budget allocations for the following financial year, and also to give an indication of other developments requiring Regional involvement. The advent of RAWP made the bidding system less significant because it proposed a formula for the allocation of resources. In the event RAWP has proved slow and difficult to implement so equity has still to be achieved. The submissions contained in District annual plans still have some effect on allocation.

A vital element of the planning process was collaboration with local authorities. Accordingly, in circular HC(77)17 issued in May 1977, the DHSS required health and local authorities, with the advice of the JCC, to set up Joint Care Planning Teams (JCPTs). Unlike the JCC these teams were to be made up of officers of the respective authorities and were to include, wherever appropriate, officers from housing, social and health services. The JCPTs could also include nominations from voluntary organisations and consumer groups. These teams were purely advisory not executive. Each JCPT advised its JCC, who in turn would make proposals to its constituent authorities. There was a possibility that the AHA or social services committees might reject the proposals and in some cases joint financing conducted under the auspices of this system has been very slow to operate. Both JCPTs and DPTs needed information to do their work effectively but found it was not always available in a useful form. This problem led, in due course, to the initiatives on improving the information systems and in particular, the work of the Körner Committee,[22] chaired by the then Vice Chairman of the South West Regional Health Authority, Edith Körner. The work of this group continued for several years and had not been concluded by 1984.

Despite the advice in circular HC(77) that membership should be kept within reasonable bounds, planning teams became and still remain somewhat cumbersome bodies which explains some of the criticism of professional advisory bodies in the Griffiths Report. Most Districts set up DPTs for the main care groups excluding the acute services (which were not seen to be suitable for joint planning in this way).

The introduction of systematic planning varied between Regions. Some of them set about planning with enthusiasm and produced their own slight amendments to the proposed system. But by 1982 there was anxiety about the system. It was cumbersome and seemed to encourage self-perpetuating talking shops, and not all Districts and Regions were working hard enough at making the system work. Accordingly, circular HC(82)6 introduced a revised planning system. This was necessary in any case, following the discontinuation of AHAs. The revised system designated the DHA as the basic planning unit and asked for five year strategic plans with annual operational plans derived from them. The advice also suggested annual reviews, but argued for less consultation because this was now deemed to be too time consuming. DHA members succeeded to the AHA places on JCCs. District Joint Care Planning Teams were set up to process the work of the District Planning Teams which continued. Where there were overlapping boundaries the District JCPT provided a forum for coordinating policies and practices between different social services departments.

The five year strategic plan was meant to give a concise summary of 'perceived needs, policies and goals' and to include references to both capital and manpower costs. In practice, the traditional split between strategic plans and operational plans continued to cause as many difficulties as it solved. If planning is deciding how tomorrow will be different from today, the means of achieving that difference will be significant in determining what to do. Strategies tend to become compromised by events and some Regions have tended to amalgamate the strategic and operational elements of each year's plan. This does not remove the need for Districts to make clear in their annual plan their overall direction which should be in line with national and regional policies. In order to make sure that Districts were conforming, the system of annual reviews was introduced in 1982 (see Chapter 2). First the Secretary of State reviews each Region and then in turn the Regions review the Districts. The Griffiths report suggested that each District should conduct similar reviews with unit teams.

Although consultation in the planning system has been reduced, Community Health Councils and Family Practitioner Committees are still involved: some have members on DPTs. The District annual plan is usually sent to district councils and county councils, but the time-scale does not always allow any meaningful consultation. The new arrangements only require formal consultation on strategic five year plans.

Although planning has come a long way since the 1974 reorganisation, problems still persist, especially at District level where the demands of everyday management tend to relegate planning to second place. Increased emphasis on accountability implies increased monitoring activity. At local level this may be undertaken in a ritualistic manner. A well articulated planning system does not guarantee results; the gap between the intention and the achievement is always difficult to bridge in any large organisation. It remains to be seen whether increased emphasis on accountability will get better results.

The remainder of the chapter discusses each care group in more detail, examining policy intentions and the success (or otherwise) of the implementation of these policies.

Primary Care

This general term covers both clients and patients. It refers to the work undertaken by general practitioners and other community staff to maintain health and, where that fails, to supporting the ill, so that wherever possible they remain out of hospital.

First the maintenance of health. This is undertaken in a general way through public health measures such as clean air regulations, proper sewage systems, environmental health inspection and through systematic surveillance of babies and children. All children can be immunised against infectious diseases, although this is not obligatory. The public health services, rather surprisingly, have not been formally integrated with the NHS except that the District Medical Officer often acts as the named officer responsible to local authorities for giving medical advice. He or she will sometimes also act as the local authority's agent in implementing certain regulations such as the transfer of someone with an infectious disease to a hospital for treatment.

Environmental health officers are employed by local authorities and operate outside the NHS. It is difficult to draw a line around the proper functions of the health service. No one would suggest that the NHS should be held responsible for bad housing or unemployment, and yet both these factors are established reasons for ill-health.

The public health programme of the last 100 years is a success story. In the United Kingdom clean water is now univerally available and cholera totally eliminated. Similarly, enteric fevers such as typhoid are rare. The steady reduction of air pollution following the Clean Air Act 1958 has reduced the incidence of chronic chest diseases in industrialised areas. A hundred years ago four babies in every ten did not survive childhood and maternal mortality was common. Now there are less than fifty maternal deaths per year. The infant mortality rate (deaths per thousand live births) is 11.0 (1982). Immunisation programmes have controlled many infectious diseases and smallpox has been totally eradicated worldwide. In the United Kingdom diphtheria, polio and scarlet fever are relatively rare and tuberculosis, measles and whooping cough much diminished. During the last 30 years, primary care services have made a concerted effort to improve health. Health visitors have had a particular responsibility for raising the general level of health and increasing attention is now being given to health promotion by health education officers.

But preventing illness is not the only responsibility of those working in primary care. Their other work relates to the care and treatment of patients in their own homes. Of one hundred patients attending a general practitioner, twelve will attend hospital as outpatients and two will become inpatients. The rest are looked after by the primary health care team headed by a general practitioner and includes a district nurse and perhaps a health visitor and social worker. The team also calls on other professionals such as a chiropodist and a physiotherapist as needed. During the last few years, there has been an increasing emphasis on the desirability of looking after patients in their own homes, not only to avoid the high cost of hospitalisation, but because the removal of the patient, particularly the very young and very old, from their own homes creates serious difficulties. Many young children become very distressed unless their parents are able to accompany them to the hospital and remain with them. Observably some elderly patients admitted to hospital become more confused. Some attempts have been made to look after even more severely ill patients at home through the Hospital-At-Home schemes.[23] It is debatable whether this is cheaper than hospitalisation and the logistic problems of the economic use of professional time are difficult to overcome.

The General Practitioner

General practice as it has developed under the NHS is almost unique in the world. In most other countries general practitioners also do some hospital medicine. In this country, although some GPs have direct access to beds of their own in local hospitals and other GPs can maintain their special interest by becoming clinical assistants to consultants, most general practice work is in the community operating from the doctors' own surgeries or from health authority-owned health centres. The original idea of the Dawson Report 1920[24] and the 1948 Labour government was that GPs should work from such health centres. In the event their development has been sporadic and by 1982 there were still only 1,050 in England. This meant that less than 20 per cent of general practitioners worked from them. Nevertheless group practices have become progressively more popular and less than 17 per cent of GPs now work single handed. The advantage of the health centre or the group practice is that team working can be developed more easily, not only allowing some degree of sub-specialisation and a proper system for deputising when one GP is off duty, but also providing more comprehensive support to the practice through attached district nurses and health visitors. Facilities for dental care, chiropody and speech therapy can also be supplied and in some cases consultants hold outpatient clinics in health centres. The average number of patients on a GP's list in the NHS is 2,146 (1981)[25] and although some GPs complain about the amount of work they are expected to undertake, patients express a high degree of satisfaction with the care and treatment provided.

District Nurses

The district nurse, is professionally supervised by the director of community nursing, who herself is accountable to the District (chief) Nursing Officer, and is usually attached to a general practice. She or he works closely with the GP, visiting patients in their own homes or seeing them for treatment in the surgery or health centre. The work covers technical nursing like wound dressings and giving medication, together with psychological support to patients and their relatives who may be worried by the patient's illness.[26]

Health Visitors

The health visitor is a highly trained nurse, a State Registered Nurse as well as a Midwife. Her work is less illness centred than that of the district nurse and she (or he) has particular responsibilities for the promotion of health. Traditionally the health visitor has spent most of her time with children, but increasingly she undertakes more work with women and the elderly. She is well placed to observe difficulties in the home and to alert other professionals to avoid crises.[26]

Other Primary Care Specialists

The *Chiropodist* is responsible for looking after people's feet – a service which is particularly important for old people. He or she can either work independently or be part of a district chiropody service, sometimes working from a clinic base and sometimes in the patient's home. The *Dental Officer* is responsible for the regular dental care of children and is closely involved with the school health service. Dental care for the elderly at clinics is now developing. Other dental care is provided by general dental practitioners operating from their own surgeries. The patient does not join a list, but enters into a contract for a course of treatment. Because of dental charges the relationship is more flexible (if more costly) than that with a general practitioner. The *Physiotherapist* is almost always attached to a hospital department, but increasingly also does domiciliary work. Most physiotherapy departments now accept referrals direct from general practitioners. Similarly, hospital-based *Occupational Therapists* are beginning to do domiciliary work. This is complicated by the fact that some other OTs are exclusively employed by Social Service departments and there is thus some risk of duplication. *Speech Therapists*, although independent professionals, take referrals from doctors. A considerable part of their work is related to the diagnosis and treatment of speech defects in children. They are also involved with a wide range of other patients particularly those with strokes or who have had a head injury and have lost the power of speech.

In addition to GP surgeries and health centres, health authorities run *Clinics* in the community either in their own premises or in rented accommodation such as church or school halls. These premises are used particularly for child developmental clinics run by specialist doctors under the supervision of the District Medical Officer. Health clinics also provide family planning services. These specialist services are described in a little more detail.

The *Child Developmental Clinic* makes sure that a child's health is supervised from the day of birth and that he or she is developing satisfactorily. Routine examinations detect hearing, speech or sight abnormalities and the child can then be referred for suitable specialist treatment. Once the child is at school he or she is examined by the school doctor at least twice during his or her school career and has more regular supervision from nurses attached to the schools. Continuous scrutiny by teachers will also help identify health or developmental problems. Towards adolescence new problems may arise such as precocious sexual activity or early addiction to smoking, drugs or solvent use and these demands can stretch the school health service beyond its present capacity.

Family Planning services are obtainable either from the GP in his own surgery or from health authority-run clinics staffed by doctors and nurses specialising in family planning work. These clinics give free contraceptive advice to men and women, married or not. They are developing a counselling service for those with sexual difficulties. This aspect of the service is also available from independent clinics. Independent agencies also provide abortion facilities for those women having difficulty because of consultant opposition or because the NHS is unable to provide an adequate service. Under the general heading of family planning male and female sterilisation clinics may also be held.

Some health authorities also provide *Well Women Clinics*. These provide a screening service for women which will include the taking of smears to check whether cancer is present in the cervix and routine breast screening. There is some debate whether these clinics are cost-effective. However, such clinics are valuable in increasing women's awareness of their bodies and helping them to carry out regular personal health checks. A similar service for men is usually only found in the private sector.

Occupational Health Services

A separate but linked example of health promotion exists in the occupational health services. Until recently there were enormous gaps in the provision of safe and healthy working environments and responsibility rested outside the NHS, being shared between a number of government departments which organised inspectorates (alkali, clean air, explosives, factories, mines and quarries and nuclear installations). These were not uniformly effective and the legislation did not require employers to inform their employees of the risks entailed in working under exposure to various dusts, fumes and chemical substances, nor to inform those who were not their employees of the risks entailed in entering such working environments. Occupational health services were set up independently by a number of firms and industries, but it was estimated that only 65 per cent of factories with 100 or fewer employees had the service of a full-time or part-time doctor. Yet for every working day lost by strikes, about ten days are lost by industrial injury or disease; most occupational accidents and diseases are preventable.

In 1948 occupational health services were not included in the remit of the NHS, and many feel this has led to their neglect and a poor understanding of their relevance to patterns of illness and health. An appointed factory doctor service was run by the Ministry of Labour, but it was only in 1973 that the Employment Medical Advisory Service came into being. This was designed to work through the Department of Employment to provide advice to ministers, employers, trade unions and other interested parties on occupational health and hygiene, and medical aspects of training and rehabilitation. Only about 120 doctors were involved in this service all over the country, the Department of Employment taking the view that engineers, chemists and other specialists rather than doctors had the expertise to assess and change the working environment. In 1972 the Robens Committee on Safety and Health at Work published its report,[27] and three years later, its full proposals were embodied in the Health and Safety at Work Act 1974, which unified responsibility for coordinating services with the Health and Safety Commission − an independent body with representatives from employers' and employees' organisations and the local authorities. The Commission has taken over the work of the Employment Medical Advisory Service and the former inspectorates and operates through the Health and Safety Executive, which employs inspectors, engineers and doctors necessary to enforce the application of the Act's provisions. Under these, all employers, employees and self-employed people (except domestic workers in private employment) are protected in the work situation and risks to the health and safety of the general public arising from work situations must be prevented. This includes control of noise, the emission of fumes, the handling of toxic materials and the risks of specific working environments. The Act operates through a series of codes of practice and requires employers to maintain safe plant and equipment, safe systems of work and premises, to arrange for adequate training, instruction and supervision, to provide facilities and arrangements for employees' welfare at work and to lay down a health and safety policy in writing and to inform employees about it. The legislation covers all staff and practitioners in the NHS for the first time, and the DHSS issues guidance from time to time relating to the particular hazards of work in the NHS.

Obviously existing occupational health services vary with different types of work setting so that the requirements of heavy manufacturing industries will differ from those of non-mechanised service enterprises.

Some firms have provided services far beyond the pre-1975 legal requirements and have delegated responsibilities to special fire and safety officers and appointed medical advisers. Nevertheless, the health and safety legislation will improve conditions overall in time, and create a better awareness of avoidable hazards. In October 1978 regulations came into force enabling safety representatives and committees to be appointed by employees. These have the power to make regular inspections and reports on conditions in the workplace and to take the advice of health and safety inspectors and make representations to the management.

Prevention of Ill-health

The maintenance of health was one of the fundamental principles of the 1946 NHS Act. But for many years the promotion of good health was left in the hands of members of the primary care team and those authorities responsible for clean water, good sewage and clean air. In 1968 the Health Education Council was established as a government-funded body and until 1973 its medical research division conducted studies on many issues including the incidence of gonorrhoea, participation in measles immunisation programmes and the causes of accidents at home. This division has now been closed down. The Health Education Council has been criticised for failing to be effective. But how is effectiveness to be judged in this area? *Prevention and Health: Everybody's Business* gave examples of successes and many of these were the result of the 19th century public health measures. Since then the immunisation programme and new drugs have helped to bring about changes in the incidence of disease. Disconcertingly, as one problem has been removed another has tended to crop up in its place: TB is now a small problem, but venereal disease is increasing; young children survive to become part of an increasingly elderly population which makes new and greater demands on services. Government policy over the last few years has done little more than state the nature of the problem and encourage authorities to do the best they can. The long drawn out campaign to introduce legislation making the wearing of seat belts compulsory could have been significantly shortened if support from the health ministers had been unequivocal. Clear evidence from other countries was largely rejected by many MPs who preferred to discuss the issue as a question of infringement of personal liberty. The substantial reduction in serious and costly accidents since the law was changed has shown how expensive the extended discussion was.

On the whole it is left to pressure groups to remind the community of the risks associated with various lifestyles and the alternatives available. As in other industrialised nations and notably the USA, promoting good health is becoming fashionable. Interest is growing in physical fitness programmes, better diet, and reducing illness-inducing activities like smoking or excessive consumption of alcohol. Health authorities were encouraged in circular HRC(74)27 to set up health education departments and there has been a renewed effort by health authorities to develop these. The terms 'Health Promotion' and 'Positive Health' are being used to give drive to these initiatives. That is needed if the fatalistic attitude of other health service staff is to be overcome. Student nurses still smoke more than their peer age group, despite receiving considerable information on the dangers of smoking. The Prevention and Health document, although a useful review, ended somewhat lamely by encouraging further discussions on ways in which people might help themselves to become fitter. It suggested that authorities should take action 'with whatever resources can be made available'. That remains the nub of the problem; too many within the NHS see health promotion as an 'extra', which can be curtailed in times of financial hardship. Governments also react in this way, which explains why in 1980 the Black Report was largely rejected by the government. Its cost implications were allowed to be made the obstacle to implementation. The Royal Commission had also drawn attention to the problems of certain social groups such as inner city populations. The DHSS's initiatives have been patchy and spasmodic as indeed they have been from other ministries.

Rather more positive government advice was contained in *Care in Action* (1981), which specifically set out the components of a local strategy for health authorities to pursue. The issues to be addressed by this strategy included a policy on smoking, the development of genetic counselling and family planning, improvement in school health services, the extension of immunisation, a programme for reducing heart disease, better health education in schools particularly covering smoking and alcohol use, nutrition and preparation for parenthood, the reduction of accidents on the road and in the home, a renewed attempt to fluoridate water supplies, and a further encouragement to maximise the contribution from voluntary, community and commercial organisations to improve health care.

Apart from the encouragement to introduce fluoridisation, successive governments have neglected prevention of dental ill-health. The

British Dental Association in a submission to the Secretary of State in 1983[28] pointed out that the escalation of dental charges amounted to dental practitioners becoming 'tax collectors for the NHS'. This was acting as a deterrent to effective dental care, particularly amongst those most at risk. As a result it was increasingly difficult to fulfil the DHSS Dental Strategy Review Group's 1981 aim of 'providing the opportunity for everyone to retain healthy functional dentition for life, by preventing what is preventable and by containing the remaining disease or deformity by the efficient use and distribution of treatment resources'.

Avoiding ill-health is economically worthwhile to our society. Despite this, governments are habitually ambivalent and the policies, where they exist, are notable more as expressions of good intentions than practical plans for action.

Acute Hospital Services

Despite the explicit objective of the NHS to promote health, the fact remains that most of its resources are devoted to the care and treatment of those who are sick and who are treated in hospital. Acute services alone absorb some 45 per cent of the total health budget. But what are the acute services? It is probably easier to define them by exception and to say that they exclude the services concerned with children and the elderly (although children and old people may become acutely ill), women having babies, the mentally ill and the physically and mentally handicapped. How is acute care provided? The patient suffers from symptoms about which the GP requires further advice or which require the special skills of the hospital consultant. This doctor has undertaken intensive training in his own specialty and has expert knowledge and, in the case of the surgeon, particular technical skills. For those patients involved in accidents or sudden collapse, referral from a GP is not necessary and they can be taken directly to the accident and emergency department of the district general hospital or to the casualty department of the local GP hospital. Most health districts have guidelines for general practitioner hospital staff and ambulance men on which cases can be handled in the local hospital and which should be transferred to the main district general hospital. In some inner city areas the district general hospital provides for both groups of patients and is effectively a substitute for the general practitioner surgery. The term 'district general hospital' was first used by the Ministry of Health Building Note No.3 in 1961 to describe a large hospital with between 400 and 800 beds, capable of providing a full range of diagnostic treatment facilities in all the major specialties and some at least of the subspecialties.

Non-emergency, but not necessary non-urgent, patients are referred by a GP to a specific consultant or group of consultants working in the appropriate specialty. The patient is given an appointment in the outpatient department which is usually held at the district general hospital. In some districts it may be at the GP hospital or health centre. The consultant or a member of his medical team examines the patient and with the help of various diagnostic procedures such as blood, urine or tissue analysis, X-ray and other methods of body and organ scanning, makes the diagnosis. This may require several visits to the hospital as an outpatient and occasionally as an inpatient treatment will be prescribed. Treatment may involve surgery, drugs, radiotherapy and physiotherapy or a combination of these. Once the patient's condition has improved sufficiently, the consultant will refer him or her back to the general practitioner. The 19th century discharge categories of 'dead', 'well' or 'relieved' are now not used, but the outcome must of course still be one or the other of these.

The cost-effectiveness of acute care is much debated. Patients are submitted to an ever increasing range of sophisticated treatments at an escalating cost and yet the outcome may well be inconclusive. Nevertheless, patients' support for these procedures is well demonstrated by the enthusiasm for raising money for high technology medical equipment. Some new procedures are very much more comfortable for the patient. For instance, patients found air encephalograms (in which air was introduced into the cavities of the brain to demonstrate the presence or otherwise of a tumour) acutely uncomfortable leaving them with a headache for several days. This has been replaced by computerised tomography using a scanner which gives the doctor more information and subjects the patient to no more discomfort than he or she would have from a routine X-ray. The introduction of fibre optics has allowed surgeons to operate inside the body, for instance in the bladder, uterus and the stomach, without having to open the patient's abdomen. One of the most notable successes of the last 20 years has been joint replacement, particularly the hip. This has been achieved by the anaesthetist and orthopaedic surgeon working together with the instrument and prosthesis maker. With improved control over anaesthetic drugs and gases the anaesthetist can now anaesthetise patients of any age without undue risk. The orthopaedic surgeon has, over the last 20 years, perfected the technique of joint replacement. As a result many elderly people previously suffering disability because of degenerating arthritic joints can be restored to active mobility.

Such success stimulates its own demand and the NHS has altogether failed to keep up so that the national waiting list for orthopaedic operations alone in March 1983 stood at 144,660. New drugs have also had remarkable effects, but there have at the same time been a few controversial failures. There is also disturbing evidence of drug-induced illness due to side effects or the prescribing of unsuitable combinations of drugs. Compared to pre-NHS days, acutely ill or injured patients now have every chance of receiving a high standard of care and treatment wherever they are in England. Despite this, problems remain.

The 1976 Priorities document was the first realistic attempt to set targets for acute care in terms other than the number of beds in a hospital. It argued that there would be slower growth of resources for this group of patients so that more could be done for the less advantaged services. The document endorsed the idea of the district general hospital providing for the usual range of medical and surgical patients as well as including a maternity unit, a psychiatric unit, a geriatric unit and children's department. Some DGHs would have full scale accident and emergency departments and some would also have ENT and eye units. A few centres would have more specialised departments, such as radiotherapy and neurosurgery. The Priorities document drew attention to the developments of recent years. First, patients' stay had gone down quite remarkably, so that the average length of stay in 1957 was 21 days and in 1977 was 13.7 days. This was due to changes in medical practice like the early ambulation of surgical patients and possibly also to such general factors as an improved home environment. Secondly, medical technology was developing too fast for the NHS to be able to cope sensibly. The Priorities document said that the pressure to adopt new techniques and equipment had to be controlled otherwise it would push up costs per case, even though patients might have to stay in hospital for a fewer number of days. No policies exist for control of the cost of the development of medical technology or 'hi-tech medicine' as it is popularly called. Each health authority has been left to work out its own solutions, so that the distribution of advanced diagnostic equipment such as computerised tomographic scanners (known as CT scanners) has been very unequal and a reflection of voluntary fund raising efforts.

Policies could be developed to encourage a more controlled expansion of medical technology and other sophisticated techniques by relying more heavily on properly regulated trials and on some form of medical audit.[29] Neither approach has yet found much direct support from government and it seems likely that health authorities will continue to hold off as best they can the seemingly insatiable demands of the acute sector, if developments for other care groups are to be achieved. The Priorities document listed the main areas of concern as being to reduce waiting times, to continue efforts to reduce unequal distribution of services, to facilitate medical advances, to improve services for the elderly and for rehabilitation. How far have these aims been pursued? There is a distinction between waiting times and waiting lists, since waiting lists represent the quantity of demand which it would be ideally reasonable to meet, whereas waiting times are something management can influence. However many patients there are on a waiting list, there should be the certainty that those there for the longest time get to the head of the queue, and when they come to hospital for consultation they are promptly dealt with. In the event, progress towards these aims has been abysmal and has stimulated an increased use of private medical facilities. Industrial unrest in 1979 and again two years later, reduced the output of some hospitals and lengthened the waiting lists considerably. Despite the Priorities document's recommendation that all urgent cases should be admitted within a month and all others within a year, many health authorities have come to accept the waiting problem as inevitable and successive governments have used it as a political weapon. By 1983 the long waiting lists were being used to discredit trade union activity within the health service and to encourage partnership with the private sector.

Children

One way of assessing health service effectiveness is to look at the health of children. To oversimplify, a healthy child means a healthy adult. Nevertheless, despite the care and attention provided by the child health services described earlier in this chapter, children are subject to sudden illness and particularly to accidents. Over 44 per cent of home accidents happen to children under 15 and similarly children are involved in 13 per cent of road accidents.[30] The regime for the acutely ill or injured child has changed remarkably in the last thirty years. Much of this has resulted from pressure applied by the parents themselves and the National Association for the Welfare of Children in Hospitals (NAWCH). Official reports, including the 1959 Platt report on the *Welfare of Children in Hospital*[31] and the Court report 1976 entitled *Fit for the Future*,[32] have also been influential. In turn, such reports were influenced by the work of enlightened paediatricians such as McCarthy and Jolly,[33] who did much to make the child's stay in hospital less of an ordeal. Most hospitals now have some facilities for parents wishing to stay with their children whilst they are in hospital. This sharing in the care of the child is not always welcomed by nursing staff and surveys by NAWCH still show that completely unrestricted visiting and reasonable facilities for parents on children's wards are by no means universal. Surgical treatment of children has changed and the routine tonsil and adenoid operation is a thing of the past. With the increasing impact of immunisation, long term inpatient care for children is now unusual and the demand for specialist children's hospitals has decreased. Concern is now centred on children in the community. The Priorities document said '1976 seems likely to be a critical year for the children's services'. Considerable criticism was expressed there and in the extensive survey published around the same time in the Court report. Both documents attacked the complacency which characterised government thinking and urged renewed efforts be made, not least to keep up with the improvements in children's health achieved in many other countries.

Over the last decade, there has been a fall in birth rate in the UK so that the under 16s represent some 22 per cent of the population in 1982 compared with 25.1 per cent in 1971. Many of these children are healthy, but an increasing number face family disruption due to the continued rise in the divorce rate. Therefore child health services have to take account of not only their physical, but their emotional and mental wellbeing. Whilst the Priorities document concentrated on specific things to be done, the Court report, a very lengthy report, was more interested in the integration of services. The Priorities document emphasised the need for further improvement in special care facilities for new-born babies. With the large scale redevelopment programme of maternity hospitals, many units have now been provided. They are run by consultant paediatricians and nurses with special training. The survival rate of low birth weight and handicapped children has increased, and this has led to the need for further care later in life. More health visitors have been needed yet not all authorities have been able to redistribute funds to do this. The Education Act 1981 requires education authorities to provide facilities for pre-school age children, but this has not yet been fully implemented. The Priorities document and *The Way Forward* emphasised the need for better secure accommodation to ensure that children were not remanded in prison. This policy has largely been achieved, although the way children's borstals and special accommodation are run has been subject to policy changes from time to time.

The Court report drew particular attention to the comparative lack of integration in services for children. For instance, general practitioners, called family doctors, are generally not fully involved in family medicine because the surveillance programme conducted by the health authorities' school health service seldom involves them directly. The justification for this is that common standards of screening and the maintenance of proper records could not be ensured if the GPs undertook these duties. Furthermore, the satisfactory surveillance of children relies increasingly on centrally held record systems. The report was also concerned with children at particular risk. 'At Risk' registers held by health authorities may not be sufficiently integrated with other records. There have been notable scandals[34] which showed that communication between health and social services departments could be improved. The implication of the Court report was that there needs to be an integrated children's service and the split of responsibility between health, social services and education leads to fragmentation and an ill-coordinated approach. The change would be difficult to implement and not surprisingly government response to the report was cool.

Maternity Services

More pregnant women than ever before are now likely to have a satisfactory outcome to their pregnancy. The perinatal mortality rate (babies dying within the first week of life together with still-births) has steadily declined and now rests at 11.3 per 1,000 births (1982). However, this is still not as good a figure as achieved by other western countries, notably Sweden. Care of the pregnant woman is one of the areas most susceptible to benefit from efforts made by professional health staff. Examination early in pregnancy by the GP and consultant obstetrician, regular supervision by the midwife and attendance at ante-natal clinics together with routine scanning and, in cases of risk, amniocentesis (the taking of a small amount of the amniotic fluid surrounding the foetus by which abnormalities such as mongolism and spina bifida can be detected) have all improved the chances of a successful birth and a healthy baby. The reduction of the number of unsatisfactory births (those with a suspect physical prognosis or just unwanted births) has been brought about by regularisation of abortion facilities following the 1967 Abortion Act. Women are now able to obtain abortions fairly easily and it is estimated that up to 3 in every 10 pregnancies are now terminated within the first few months.[35]

Some would argue that not all the changes are good for the mother. For instance, hospitalisation of almost all births may have improved the chances of the baby and its mother, but even this evidence is somewhat confusing, given the good results found in Holland where, alone in Europe, there is still a relatively high domiciliary delivery rate. Nevertheless, the recommendations of the Cranbrook report[36] in 1959 which advocated the greater hospitalisation of mothers in labour and of the Peel report[37] in 1970 which emphasised the need for an integrated approach to maternal care, have resulted directly and indirectly in the present hospital delivery rate of around 98 per cent. With this has come greater pressure to reduce the institutional regime of the maternal confinement. New – and possibly very old – theories about how best to be delivered in more homely settings with the attendance of the father at the birth, have helped to normalise delivery and reduce the institutional atmosphere.[38] It seems unlikely that there will be a large scale return to home confinements, not least because GPs and domiciliary midwives, lacking experience of the home delivery, are becoming increasingly reluctant to undertake them.

The Cranbrook report was critical of the existing standards which put mothers and their babies unnecessarily at risk. It proposed that at least 70 per cent of mothers should be delivered in hospital. The length of stay was assumed to be ten days, requiring 0.58 beds per 1,000 population on the projected population figures for 1975. The 1962 plan accepted this recommendation unequivocally and for the next 20 years maternity hospital buildings were gradually renewed throughout the country. With the decline in the birth rate and the reduction in the length of stay to around six days, some areas then found they had too many beds. This was not entirely the result of a policy change, so much as a change in obstetrics and midwifery practice. The introduction of new procedures, such as scanning and amniocentesis has tended to direct the mother to the district general hospital maternity unit and ante-natal clinic at least at some point in her pregnancy and, as a result, the number of GPs and community midwives who feel able to undertake deliveries has declined.

Despite the improvement in facilities for pregnant women, comparative statistics show that the UK has been trailing behind other countries in such matters as perinatal mortality. The Short report of 1980 (a Select Committee report)[39] examined this further and encouraged the government not to reduce their concern with the improvement of maternity services. Since the 1950s, doctors themselves have undertaken reviews of their practice through triennial confidential enquiries into maternal deaths. These reviews have shown that around half of all maternal deaths need not have happened. Social factors contribute to risk in pregnancy and the Black report on inequalities[40] demonstrated that a deprived mother was less likely to seek care and was consequently more likely to put her own health and that of her baby in jeopardy. Maternal deaths in the 1960s amongst occupational class V mothers were double that of class I and II. This pattern still holds true.

The Mentally Handicapped

Despite improved care of mothers and babies during pregnancy and birth, some babies are born with mental handicap or subsequently develop this impairment. Classification of the numbers of mentally handicapped people is fraught with problems of description. It has been customary to rely heavily on intelligence quotient (IQ) so that those registered under 50 are called severely handicapped and those between 50 and 70 mildly handicapped. The IQ measure is not without its critics and it is not always a good indicator of the needs of a mentally handicapped person. Accordingly, this has led to attempts to define mentally handicapped people in terms of the level of their dependency on others, but even this has proved to be inexact. It is repeatedly found that highly dependent mentally handicapped people who were institutionalised can make radical progress in a different environment, becoming much more capable than even optimistic professional staff would have predicted.

There are three to four severely handicapped people per thousand in the 15-19 age group. Mental handicap is not an identifiable disease; it is the result of malfunction during pregnancy, injury at birth, or injury subsequently by accident, infection, drugs or a developing degenerative condition. The management of such people has to take account of this variety of causes. Interestingly, the name of the condition has troubled every generation and reflects the changing attitude of society to the problem. From the 'idiots' of the late 19th century the descriptive and legal terms have included 'deficiency', 'subnormality' and now 'mental handicap'. In other countries the present preferred term is 'mental retardation'. With the changes of name, have come changed attitudes and the last 15 years have been particularly significant for the amount of discussion on how best to look after mentally handicapped people. But despite this, the record of achievement has not been particularly impressive. Some progress is being made and a few health authorities and social services departments are pursuing increasingly radical policies, particularly those aimed at deinstitutionalising the service. There are, however, still around 40,000 mentally handicapped people remaining in hospital.

Government pressure has focused on the discharge of mentally handicapped children from long term hospital care,[41] but this has been the easiest problem to solve, given the considerable support available to families. As well as health visitors and other specialist staff, an increasing number of opportunity groups are being established. These are pre-school groups for the handicapped (not necessarily mentally handicapped). Attempts to integrate mentally handicapped children in ordinary schools will have limited success so special schools will continue to fulfil most of this need. Handicapped children are entitled to education up to the age of 19 although not all education authorities fulfil their obligations in this respect. After 19, the adult training centre and the sheltered workshop may give mentally handicapped people a place to go during the day. Within some large mental handicap hospitals similar opportunities for work exist, but many mentally handicapped people spend their day without much occupation or diversion.

Mental handicap has gradually attracted more attention from professional health services staff. Amongst administrators at least it is no longer seen as a low prestige area of work. This was first stimulated by the recurring scandals arising from lack of appropriate care, starting with the Ely Hospital affair of 1969[42] and Pauline Morris' study *Put Away*[43] the same year. The most significant policy document was *Better Services for the Mentally Handicapped* (1971),[44] which could almost be said to be a mentally handicapped people's charter. The long term aims were to provide a more satisfactory environment for them, whether this was at home, in a hospital or in a residential home. The traditional segregation from society was deplored; health, social services and educational authorities were encouraged to work together to provide an integrated, readily accessible service. Every effort was to be made to support families of mentally handicapped people. The Priorities document endorsed these policy aims and proposed considerable growth in the number of local authority training centres and residential homes. Staffing ratios in hospitals were to be increased and would help improve the standards. In 1975 the National Development

Group was set up to lead the way to these better standards. Their regular reports were important in maintaining government commitment. Despite this the Group was disbanded in 1980, but not before the government had published a review of the progress since the *Better Services* document. In fact progress had been disappointing. One of the reasons for this was the conflict between professionals about the best way of providing care. Some staff are convinced that the increasing emphasis on community care is wrong, both for the community who could feel threatened by mentally handicapped people in their midst, and for the mentally handicapped people themselves who could be discriminated against and would lose the access to those facilities provided as a matter of course in mental handicap hospitals. The Jay report[45] published in 1979 fanned the flames of disagreement by suggesting that the training of nurses in mental handicap was largely inappropriate and a less clinically-based training would be better. In the event, faced with this professional controversy and because the financial implications were considerable, the government did not support the Jay recommendations.

After ten years of discussion the policy of discharging mentally handicapped people into the community remains. This has been made easier now that the money can be provided by joint finance and since collaboration with voluntary bodies is encouraged. In 1983, the government was offering financial incentives to discharge long-stay mentally handicapped children from hospital and *Care in the Community* offered similar encouragement in an attempt to resettle adult mentally handicapped people. The longer term policy is still undecided. Should the government transfer the responsibility for all mentally handicapped people to social services, or indeed to the voluntary sector? Any government will find it politically advisable to be sensitive to the care and rights of mentally handicapped people. Policies may be published, but experience has shown that their achievement is not thereby guaranteed.

The Physically Disabled

Another relatively small group of people requiring considerable support from the health service is the physically disabled. This broad label covers people with a variety of conditions. Disablement may be due to injury, particularly the results of a road accident, or infectious or degenerative disease, or sudden medical emergencies such as a stroke.

The demands made by a disabled person will naturally vary according to his or her problem. At the most severe level the disabled person will need complete medical and nursing care in a hospital. All too often this care is provided in unsuitable accommodation: an acute ward where the high level of turnover is not suitable for someone having to live there for a long period. Or worse still, for a younger disabled person, is life in a ward of elderly patients, some of whom may be confused.

Unfortunately many health professionals tend to underestimate the potential for improvement in heavily disabled people, particularly those with head injuries, those with multiple sclerosis and stroke victims. Without an early and coordinated attempt to estimate the rehabilitative potential or the appropriate level of alleviation, the patient will not only fail to improve, but will find himself developing further problems.

Following the passing of the *Chronically Sick and Disabled Persons Act* 1970,[46] health authorities started to develop special units for the younger disabled. But the policy seemed to run out of steam and there are still less than 2000 places in purpose-built hospital units. This means that many patients do not benefit from appropriate care. The Priorities document gave muted support to the provision of such hospital units, although it pressed strongly for a special spinal injuries unit for the south of England to relieve pressure on the unit at Stoke Mandeville Hospital. A new spinal injuries unit opened at Odstock Hospital, Salisbury, in 1984. Otherwise emphasis has been on maintaining the physically handicapped in the community or in homes provided by the voluntary sector.

Disabled people who can continue living outside hospital may be supported usefully by cash benefits and visits from support staff. The attendance allowance is a benefit which subsidises the cost of someone giving long-term physical assistance. Social services and health authorities are empowered to lend or give the disabled person an extensive array of physical aids to daily living. House adaptations can also be provided free of charge. Nevertheless, the disabled person may still find getting around difficult and public buildings have not yet been adapted as thoroughly as the 1970 Act suggested. Work can be difficult to find for disabled people, particularly in a time of high unemployment. Sheltered working conditions are relatively limited and often provide very tedious work for the physically handicapped person of normal intelligence. Physically handicapped people, unlike those with mental handicap, are able to speak for themselves, and pressure groups such as the Disablement Income Group and the Disabled Drivers' Association continue to put pressure on government and social services and health authorities. Voluntary bodies also provide considerable support, both in the provision of residential accommodation and in advocacy for disabled people's needs.

The Mentally Ill

It could be said that the physically disabled do better than the mentally ill because their condition does not normally attract the same amount of stigma. Mental disorders still frighten many people and primitive reactions to madness underlie their responses.

Large mental illness hospitals isolated from the community are still found in many health districts. The 1962 plan envisaged the gradual closure of these hospitals, most of which were built following the asylum legislation of the second half of the 19th century. Although there has been a remarkable reduction in the size of such hospitals over the last ten years, the institutions still exist and will continue to do so, unless there is a substantial change in the allocation of capital funds to mental illness to allow new smaller units to be built. Opinion is divided as to whether this is the best policy.

Mental disorder, unlike much mental handicap, is an illness. Do patients fare better left at home supported by visiting specialist staff or do they recover more quickly if admitted to a hospital away from the environment which may have contributed to their illness? If it is the latter, should this be a small local unit reasonably accessible to its own community or is it better to use the larger hospital which because of its size can provide a wider range of therapeutic regimes? Such questions remain largely unresolved and, whilst this continues, large mental illness hospitals seem likely to remain. Nevertheless, day care continues to develop and can be particularly valuable in the support of those chronically ill people whose symptoms are an irritant to their families rather than a cause of total family disruption. Day care is also more likely to be useful in looking after the elderly mentally ill. Whether senile dementia is really a classifiable condition or merely a useful generalisation for a range of behaviour problems found in old people is not clear. Admitting a patient to hospital with episodes of confusion often increases their disorientation, and although support in their own homes surrounded by their own family and possessions is more humane, the strain on families should not be underestimated.

As with the mentally handicapped, the problem of definition is considerable. Leaving aside those radical views which hold that it is not people who are ill but society,[47] opinion still differs about the nature of mental illness. Traditionally, patients are categorised into two main groups: the psychotic and the neurotic (and the term neurotic is used here rather more technically than in common language). Those suffering from psychosis seem to others to have a poor perception of reality; they may be convinced that they are right and everyone else is wrong and their delusions may be consequently bizarre. The person with neurosis characteristically has a view of reality which most other people would share, but has a problem in coping and is subject to a high level of anxiety and distress, which can be sufficiently disabling to require professional support in or out of hospital. Psychosis is apparently found in all populations and social cultures and does not appear to be related to class. Neurosis, however, is more specifically related to social conditions and class.

Treatment for the mentally ill varies even for the same conditions. Some psychiatrists, psychologists and nurses feel that the encouragement of self help through group therapy is both humane and effective,[48] while others rely more on helping the patient to cope through drugs and in some cases electroconvulsive therapy (ECT). Psychotherapy demands a long and time-consuming interaction with the patient. It is rarely provided within the NHS because of a lack of resources as well as professional doubts about its efficacy. The treatment of the mentally ill depends on satisfactory team working. The doctor, the clinical psychologist, the nurse, the social worker, the occupational therapist and others need to agree a treatment plan to get the best results. For many patients their illness will be a recurring event. In order to take the stigma out of these episodes of ill health the DHSS's policy has been to encourage the development of community support, thus avoiding hospital admission. But where this is necessary, stigma may be reduced if admission is to a mental illness unit in a new district general hospital.

Despite the uncertainty about therapeutic methods the last twenty-five years have seen considerable improvements. In the mid-1950s there were over 150,000 people in mental illness hospitals. The consequent overcrowding meant that standards were very low and wards with over 60 patients were commonplace. The 1959 Mental Health Act[49] did a great deal to reduce the numbers compulsorily admitted to hospital and this, together with developments in drug therapy, started a gradual reduction in hospital numbers. The 1962 Plan optimistically predicted the closure of a substantial number of the older isolated mental illness hospitals, to be replaced by smaller units attached to DGHs.

In 1975 a White Paper entitled *Better Services for the Mentally Ill*[50] set out the government's long term policies. These were first, that more facilities would be provided within the community to keep the mentally ill out of hospital, and consequently, day hospitals, sheltered work and adequate home support all needed to be expanded. Secondly, if people became ill enough for hospital they should be admitted wherever possible to either the local DGH or, if old and mentally infirm, to the local community hospital. Thirdly, staffing ratios were to be improved, particularly medical, nursing and social work staff. Fourthly, where older hospitals remained, renewed attempts should be made to improve standards. The Priorities document supported these aspirations, but the Royal Commission in 1979 said the policies were ambiguous, particularly regarding the closure of old mental illness hospitals. The Royal Commission said that realistically any government would have to accept that most mental illness hospitals would remain open for the rest of the century at least. Policy, therefore, should centre on providing a balanced service within which these hospitals could play a part. Financial stringency at the beginning of the 1980s forced many health authorities to review their strategies for the mentally ill. Increasingly, agency agreements between authorities whereby one provides services for another, were causing difficulties. So government policies may well encourage authorities to be more self-sufficient. As well as the allocation of resources, the internal organisation of the psychiatric services has worried successive governments. The Nodder report (1980)[51] supported the consensus team approach, but was critical of the lack of direction shown by many of these teams. A more structured approach with annual objectives and routine monitoring of achievement was advocated. The discussion leading to the 1982 reorganisation submerged most of these proposals, but in some cases unit management teams set up after 1982 are operating along the lines suggested by Nodder.

Poor results may arise because objectives are poorly formulated, but this is not the case with secure units. The Priorities document proposed a secure unit for each Region and allocated capital monies there and then. Eight years later most of these have not been built, either because of staff opposition or because of failure to agree on the type of patient who should be accommodated there. Although the Mental Health Act 1983[52] gave health authorities greater responsibilities for safe-guarding the rights of their patients, progress in the care of the mentally ill remains much too slow: many of the principles set out in the 1975 *Better Services* document have still not been implemented. This may be because the range of problems has diffused a clear sense of direction. Alcohol and drug abuse are causing increasing illness, but more pressing than these are the demands being made by the elderly mentally ill, whose numbers will continue to increase with their proportionate increase in the population during the next decade.

The Elderly

The largest broad category of patients is the elderly. About 14 per cent of the population is aged 65 and over. This proportion is expected to decline, although there will still be a rise in the number of the very old (those over 75). These statistics reflect steady improvements in child health since the beginning of the century, rather than an increasing life expectancy in the elderly themselves. Broadly speaking, the longer you live, the longer you live. However, the quality of life in physical terms diminishes and those over 75 are ten times more likely to see their general practitioner over a year than the rest of the adult population. Old age brings many symptoms, some due to physical degeneration such as deafness, blindness and arthritis, some because of mental incapacity. Ironically the mental confusion can be increased by the intervention of professional staff, so that an elderly person admitted to a geriatric assessment unit may at first be more disoriented than before admission. Opinion is divided as to how much treatment, as opposed to care, should be given to the very old. Geriatricians anxious to be given the status accorded to their general physician colleagues, may increasingly be tempted to submit their patients to a battery of clinical investigations. On the other hand, before geriatricians were appointed, the passiveness of care and lack of treatment given in many hospitals for the elderly resembled conditions when they were still work-houses. A balance between active intervention and letting life take its course has to be found.

Specialist care of old people is a phenomenon of the post-war era. Geriatricians attempt to see the patient as a whole person, concentrating on their environment as well as their health. Problems all too often arise in the discharge of an elderly person because insufficient account is taken of their home circumstances. Most elderly people in hospital are not in the care of the geriatrician, but have been referred to other specialists. Only 20 per cent of district general hospitals have specialist geriatric units.

The proportion of old people in hospital or residential accommodation is still small. Remaining at home, old people require increasing support from health and social services and in times of financial stringency, it is often these support services which are cut first. However incapacitated they may be, many elderly people wish to remain at home and may endure considerable physical and financial hardship to do so. Professional staff in the NHS know that more could be done and the elderly have become an increasingly important priority group. The diffuseness of the problem, however, makes coherent planning difficult. The need for specific plans for the elderly was recognised in the 1962 Plan which said that every DGH should have an active geriatric unit where elderly patients could be assessed, even those who would subsequently need long term care. The Priorities document reported that it had been DHSS policy for some time to have 50 per cent of geriatric beds provided in a DGH. This has never been achieved and the 1980 Future Patterns paper accepted 30 per cent as an interim target. Even these numbers have failed to materialise in many Districts. The Priorities document thought that ten beds per 1000 population over 65 was a reasonable guideline. Some regions have suggested a lower figure. In 1978 the government brought out a consultative document called *A Happier Old Age*,[53] which stressed the need to keep elderly people in the community for as long as possible, giving them support through home helps, district nurses, day centres and meals on wheels. It said voluntary bodies should be encouraged to help in these tasks. The Royal Commission a year later supported this general view, but noted that geriatrics should remain part of the mainstream of medicine if a fully integrated service was to be provided. More active research into the problems of the elderly was encouraged.

In a consultation paper issued in 1980 called *The Future Pattern of Hospital Provision in England*[54] the idea of an NHS elderly nursing home as an alternative to hospital was discussed, but it took until 1984 to set one up.[55] The advantages were seen as a less institutional atmosphere and less overall running costs. As part of the encouragement of partnership between the public and private sectors the 1982 Conservative government gave considerable emphasis to supporting the private sector by increasing social security benefits to encourage elderly people to remain in such homes, rather than be admitted to NHS beds. The 1981 White Paper *Growing Older*,[56] did little more than support the general direction policies had been taking for over a decade. Put simply these policies supported the maintenance of elderly people in the community as long as possible. When illness necessitated hospital admission, this should be to an acute assessment unit which had been shown to reduce the overall length of stay. Only for the most dependent should longer term hospital care be contemplated. There is evidence that health authorities have yet to appreciate the significance of the growing numbers of elderly. More recently the government has been repeatedly criticised for not allocating sufficient resources to keep up with the increase in the demands from the elderly.

This chapter has endeavoured to show how plans and policies for patients have been developed over the last 20 years. It has to be said, however, that many of the policies have been little more than statements of good intent. Only the 1976 Priorities document made a real attempt to match policies with resources and this was quickly stifled by the worsening economic climate of the late 1970s. Policies of the early 1980s have concentrated on alternatives to direct provision by the NHS.

Notes

1. Ministry of Health. *Report of the Committee of Enquiry into the Cost of the National Health Service*. (Guillebaud Report), HMSO, London, 1956 (Cmnd. 9663).
2. Ministry of Health. *A Hospital Plan for England and Wales*, HMSO, London, 1962 (Cmnd. 1604).
3. Ibid., p. iii, para. 1.
4. Ministry of Health. *The Hospital Building Programme. A Revision of the Hospital Plan for England and Wales*, HMSO, London, 1966.
5. Central Health Services Council. *The Functions of the District General Hospital* (Bonham-Carter Report), HMSO, London, 1969.
6. DHSS. Circular HSC(15)75. *Community Hospitals*.
7. Ministry of Health. *Health and Welfare – the Development of Community Care*, HMSO, London, 1963.
8. DHSS. *Priorities for Health and Personal Social Services in England*. A Consultative Document, HMSO, London, 1976.
9. Ibid., p. iii, para. 4.
10. DHSS. *The Way Forward*, HMSO, London, 1977.
11. DHSS. *Sharing Resources for Health in England*. Report of the Resource Allocation Working Party (RAWP), HMSO, London, 1976.
12. DHSS. Circular HC(76)18/LAC(76)6. *Joint Care Planning: Health and Local Authorities*.
13. DHSS. Circular HC(77)17/LAC(77)10. *Joint Care Planning: Health and Local Authorities*.
14. DHSS. *Prevention and Health: Everybody's Business*. A Consultative Document, HMSO, London, 1976.
15. DHSS. *Hospital Services. The Future Pattern of Hospital Provision in England*. A Consultative Document, HMSO, London, 1980.

16. DHSS. *Care in Action – A Handbook of Policies and Priorities for the Health and Personal Social Services in England*, HMSO, London, 1981.

17. DHSS. *Care in the Community*, HMSO, London, 1981. But see also Circular HC(83)6/LAC(83)5 on, *Care in the Community and Joint Finance*.

18. DHSS. *Report of the Working Group on Inequalities in Health* (Black Report), HMSO, London, 1980.

19. DHSS. *The NHS Management Inquiry* (Griffiths Report), see Chapter 1, note 40 for publication history.

20. DHSS. *Guide to Planning in the National Health Service*, HMSO, London, 1975.

21. DHSS. *NHS Planning System*, HMSO, London, 1976.

22. DHSS. *Steering Group on Health Services Information* (Chairman Mrs Edith Körner). Various reports from 1976 onwards.

23. Hospital-at-Home was developed in France. See Cang, S. Lancet, i, 1977, 742. for a description.

24. Ministry of Health. *Interim Report of the Future Provision of Medical and Allied Services*, (Dawson Report), HMSO, London, 1920.

25. Quoted from DHSS sources in *General Practice – A British Success*, BMA – General Medical Services Committee, London, 1983.

26. For a more detailed account of these two branches of nursing see *Nursing, Midwifery and Health Visiting since 1900*, edited by Allan and Jolley, Faber & Faber, London, 1982.

27. *Safety and Health at Work*. Report of the Committee 1970–72, HMSO, London, 1972 (Cmnd 5034).

28. British Dental Association. *NHS Dental Treatment. What it costs and how the cost has risen*, BDA, London, 1983.

29. For a discussion of some of the issues surrounding high technology medicine see *The Image and the Reality* by Barbara Stocking and S. Morrison, O.U.P. for the Nuffield Provincial Hospitals Trust, Oxford, 1978.

30. These figures need treating with caution. The home accidents represent hospital-treated non-fatal accidents calculated from a sample of 20 hospitals. The road accidents are calculated from police-reported road accidents.

31. Ministry of Health. Central Health Services Council. *The Welfare of Children in Hospital* (Platt Report), HMSO, London, 1959.

32. DHSS. Committee on Child Health Services. *Fit for the Future* (Court Report), HMSO, London, 1976 (Cmnd 6684).

33. McCarthy developed a mother and child unit at Amersham General Hospital in the 1950s. Jolly, first at Plymouth and then at the Charing Cross Hospital, London was a leading paediatrician.

34. The Maria Colwell case in the mid-1970s emphasised the dilemma of the health and social services in making decisions about where a child should be maintained. In this case the child died from ill-treatment and the authorities were much criticised for not taking her into care.

35. There were 140,000 legal abortions in 1981 against a birth rate of 730,000 (OPCS statistics). Since then the birth rate has continued to decline and the abortion rate has increased. Not all abortions are officially registered.

36. Ministry of Health. *Report of the Maternity Services Committee* (Cranbrook Report), HMSO, London, 1959.

37. DHSS. Central Health Services Council. *Domiciliary Midwifery and Maternity Bed Needs* (Peel Report), HMSO, London, 1970.

38. Notably F. LeVoyer, *Birth without Violence*, Wildwood House, London, 1974 and M. Odent, *Entering the World: the demedicalisation of childbirth*, Marion Boyars, London, 1983.

39. Reply to the Second Report from the Social Services Committee, *Report*

on Perinatal and Neonatal Mortality (Short Report), HMSO, London, 1980 (Cmnd 8084).

40. Op. cit. as published by Penguin Books 1982, see p. 82, Table 16.

41. DHSS. Circular HC(83)21/LAC(83)15. *Helping to Get Mentally Handicapped Children Out of Mental Handicap Hospitals*, 1983.

42. DHSS. *Report of the Committee of Enquiry into Allegations of Ill-Treatment of Patients and Other Irregularities at Ely Hospital, Cardiff.* (Howe Report), HMSO, London, 1969 (Cmnd 3795).

43. Pauline Morris, *Put Away*, Routledge & Kegan Paul, London, 1969.

44. DHSS and Welsh Office. *Better Services for the Mentally Handicapped*, HMSO, London, 1971 (Cmnd 4683).

45. DHSS. *Committee of Enquiry into Mental Handicap Nursing and Care* (Jay Report), HMSO, London, 1979 (Cmnd 7468).

46. *Chronically Ill and Disabled Persons Act* 1970, HMSO, London. See also Circular HM(70)52.

47. Notably T. Szasz, *The Myth of Mental Illness*, Harper and Row, New York, 1976. See also Illich, *The Limits to Medicine*, Penguin Books, Harmondsworth, 1977.

48. Notably at Dingleton Hospital, Melrose, Scotland, described in Jones, M., *The Process of Change*, Routledge & Kegan Paul, London, 1982.

49. *Mental Health Act 1959*, HMSO, London, 1959.

50. DHSS. *Better Services for the Mentally Ill*, HMSO, London, 1975 (Cmnd 6233).

51. DHSS. *Organisational and Management Problems of Mental Illness Hospitals.* (Nodder Report), HMSO, London, 1980.

52. *Mental Health Act 1983*, HMSO, London, 1983.

53. DHSS. *A Happier Old Age*, HMSO, London, 1978.

54. DHSS. Hospital Services: *The Future Pattern of Hospital Provision in England.* A Consultation Paper, May 1980.

55. In Portsmouth Health District. See description in *Health and Social Services J.*, 21.7.83.

56. DHSS. *Growing Older*, HMSO, London, 1981 (Cmnd 8173).

8 DOCTORS

This chapter is concerned with the professional organisation of doctors, their education and training, their distribution, their working arrangements in the NHS and their remuneration. The development of medicine as a scientifically-based understanding of health and disease has depended on the pace of discoveries in the natural sciences. The last 100 years have seen the most rapid changes, although important landmarks date earlier than that.

Professional Organisations

Before 1700 the medical profession was firmly divided into three groups: the physicians, surgeons and apothecaries. The physicians had the highest status, and the Royal College of Physicians of London was founded in 1518. The members were graduates of Oxford and Cambridge universities, who had received religious and classical education, and subsequently often studied medical subjects in European universities. The surgeons were not scholars but craftsmen organised in a guild that was associated with the barbers, and they were licensed to perform the small range of procedures that could be carried out on unanaesthetised patients. Apothecaries were tradesmen who, from 1617 were licensed by the Society of Apothecaries to sell drugs prescribed by physicians. Until 1700 treatment was essentially carried out in the patients' homes. However, the position changed between 1700 and about 1850, partly because that period saw the rise of the great voluntary hospitals which provided the setting for developments in surgery; in comparison, the physicians hardly advanced their techniques and abilities. The prestige of surgeons rose and in 1745 the Company of Surgeons was founded, cementing their independence from the barbers and enabling educational standards to improve; by 1800 the Company had become the Royal College of Surgeons of England.

Apothecaries also advanced, and by 1703 they were entitled to see patients and prescribe medicines themselves. The result was that they became the 'general practitioners' for the middle classes and the poor. The Apothecaries Act of 1815 gave the Society of Apothecaries the right to license those who had served a five year apprenticeship and passed examinations, and some physicians took this qualification as well. As the voluntary hospitals were closed to these practitioners and only employed the services of those recognised by the Royal Colleges, the distinction between consultants and general practitioners became established. The Society of Apothecaries pioneered improvements in the standard of education and in raising the status of practitioners far more than the universities or Royal Colleges did – from 1842 to 1844 sixteen practitioners were licensed by the universities of Oxford and Cambridge, thirty-seven by the Royal College of Physicians, and 953 by the Society of Apothecaries. Despite this success, unqualified practitioners flourished (the 1841 census showed over 30,000 doctors, while the first Medical Directory published in 1845 listed only 11,000 qualified practitioners), and demand for a single licensing authority and a single professional qualification permitting practice in any branch of the profession arose. The strongest pressure for such a licence came from the Provincial Medical and Surgical Association. This body was founded in Worcester in 1832, and drew so much support that by 1855 it had changed its name to the British Medical Association. The campaign resulted in the passing of the Medical Act in 1858, which created the General Council of Medical Education and Registration.[1] It is now called the General Medical Council (GMC) and has fifty members representing the Royal Colleges, the universities, the Crown and the profession at large. Their duty is to maintain a register of practitioners licensed by recognised authorities, and to supervise the educational standards of training institutions. In practice the GMC rely on medical schools to maintain standards in undergraduate training, and on the Royal Colleges for postgraduate and specialist training. Health Authorities are constantly reminded of the power of the Royal Colleges to remove training approval from hospital posts and this threatened sanction has done much to improve standards of training and also to support facilities such as medical libraries.

Following the 1975 Merrison Report[2] the GMC constitution was changed and greater attention has since been paid to registration matters, particularly of overseas doctors, who make up over 30 per cent of hospital medical staff. Such doctors are given limited registration for up to five years and their admittance to full registration relies on satisfactory reports of their work.

The GMC are also concerned with disciplinary matters and have the power to remove a doctor from the Medical Register in cases of serious professional misconduct such as criminal convictions which would make it undesirable to continue in practice.

Other medical corporations to have been established include the Royal College of Obstetricians and Gynaecologists (1929), the Royal College of General Practitioners (1952), the Royal College of Pathologists (1962) and the Royal College of Psychiatrists (1971).

The Royal Colleges and other medical corporations are not trade unions for doctors, but bodies mainly concerned with post-registration training and development, and until comparatively recently they only represented the elite specialties of the profession. The British Medical Association (BMA) emerged as the spokesman for the 'underdog' general practitioners. For example, it threatened Lloyd George's government with destruction of the National Health Insurance Scheme through the refusal of the GPs' cooperation just as the scheme was about to be implemented. The opposition was dropped in 1912 when the government agreed to the demand for a higher rate of remuneration for GPs. Before that time the outpatient departments and dispensaries of the voluntary hospitals provided treatment subsidised by the charitable organisations, and thus represented an alternative source of treatment for people which might be chosen instead of going to a general practitioner who contracted to work for a friendly society, if private treatment could not be afforded. But the 1911 Act had the effect of greatly increasing the numbers of people entitled to medical benefit through membership of the approved societies, and hence safeguarded the level of GPs' incomes under the National Health Insurance Scheme. The rivalry between the GPs and the hospital doctors was considerable and the BMA set out the terms of their relationships in a code of ethics which made the GP responsible for his patients while the specialists could be consulted for opinion and advice on diagnosis and treatment. This enabled GPs to maintain their list of patients without the fear that if any of them were referred to a hospital doctor, he would take them over; to the present day hospital doctors do not have a list of registered patients for whom they assume continuing responsibility.

Other bodies have emerged to protect doctors' interests, including the Junior Hospital Doctors' Association (5,500 members), the Hospital Consultants' and Specialists' Association (5,000 members) and the Medical Practitioners Union (about 4,000 members), but the BMA (with a membership of about 50,000 in the UK) is still regarded as the foremost and legitimate spokesman for all doctors, whether or not they are members. Its role in the setting up of the NHS in the 1940s has been described in Chapter 1, and since that time its internal organisation has been modified such that it mirrors the structure of the NHS – hospital doctors are represented in the BMA by its Central Committee for Hospital Medical Services, while GPs are separately represented by its General Medical Services Committee. The constituents of these two committees are the Local Medical Committees and Regional Committees for Hospital Medical Staffs, on which doctors working in the NHS are represented. The BMA leadership has not always been regarded by individual doctors as being in touch with their interests and there have been a number of occasions when it has been unable publicly to present a convincing view of the profession's position. One factor which may contribute to this impression is that there are three separate bodies (or sets of bodies) acting for the profession – the medical corporations for professional representation, the GMC for discipline and self-regulation, and the BMA for pay negotiations.

Medical Education

The training of doctors involves a large element of practical experience and in the past, students were apprenticed to physicians, surgeons and apothecaries, the university part of their training representing a relatively small element. The balance has now altered, although this tradition has had a substantial influence on the style of undergraduate curricula, and postgraduate education is still mainly in the hands of the professional organisations rather than the universities. By 1858 there were eleven medical schools in London and at least ten in the provinces apart from the universities of Oxford and Cambridge. By 1914 all except four of the present provincial university medical schools were open. Currently there are thirty-one undergraduate medical schools in the UK (see Figure 23).

Before the First World War, teaching of clinical subjects was provided by physicians and surgeons who, although in private practice gave their services to the hospitals where students were apprenticed as clerks and dressers for short periods. Pre-clinical subjects were taught by doctors engaged in clinical work who often did not specialise in these subjects. The Haldane report published in 1912 strongly criticised these features and recommended there should be full-time clinical teachers of university status and that units of medicine and surgery under clinicians with professorial status should organise and provide the clinical teaching. It was not until the 1920s however, that things

Figure 23 *Medical Schools in the United Kingdom*

Medicine was being taught in several of these centres before a medical school was formally established or incorporated into an existing university.

ENGLAND		LONDON	
Birmingham	1828	Charing Cross	1834
Bristol	1833	Guy's	1769
Cambridge	14th century	King's College	1831
Leeds	1831	London	1785
Leicester	1975	Middlesex	1835
Liverpool	1834	Royal Free	1874
Manchester	1814	St. Bartholemew's	1726
Newcastle	1834	St. George's	1831
Nottingham	1970	St. Mary's	1854
Oxford	14th century	St. Thomas's	1723
Sheffield	1828	University College	1828
Southampton	1971	Westminster	1834

WALES		SCOTLAND	
Welsh National		Aberdeen	1840
School of Medicine	1931	Dundee	1898
		Edinburgh	1726
		Glasgow	1714
		St. Andrew's	1898

NORTHERN IRELAND
Belfast   1849

began to change, and this was partly due to the establishment of the University Grants Committee which was given responsibility for the financing of the universities. The medical schools were becoming steadily more dependent on the universities for funds. Research and specialisation extended as a result, but by 1944 the idea of full-time specialist units had not really been implemented and there were only seven full-time chairs in medicine, four in surgery and two in obstetrics. In that year, the Inter-departmental Committee on Medical Schools published its report (the Goodenough report).[3] It reaffirmed the main points of the Haldane report and proposed full-time professorial units in obstetrics and gynaecology as well as in medicine and surgery. It suggested premedical studies should be started by potential medical students at secondary school and continued at medical school, and that after qualification, one year of pre-registration hospital work under supervision should provide the necessary practical experience before a newly qualified doctor could work on his own.

The pattern of undergraduate education was further investigated by a Royal Commission chaired by Lord Todd, from 1965 to 1968.[4] At that time students with high passes in biology, chemistry and physics 'A' level examinations were admitted to medical schools for five terms of pre-clinical instruction which basically covered anatomy, physiology and biochemistry. After examination the students then studied for three more years, partly in the hospital wards and partly in formal lectures. The subjects included medicine, surgery and sometimes psychiatry. They took examinations in these subjects too before obtaining their qualifying degree (MB, BS or MB, ChB or MB, BChir),[5] and then had to spend one further year in approved training posts as house officers before being registered. There was subsequently no compulsory further education, although if a junior doctor wanted to advance his career in certain specialties, he would have to take further instruction and examination, leading to Membership of the Royal College of Physicians (MRCP) or Fellowship of the Royal College of Surgeons (FRCS), for example.

The Todd report is a comprehensive document that questioned the basic assumptions on which medical education had been based, and made several radical recommendations about its future organisation. It suggested that the undergraduate curriculum should be broad and flexible, to include sociological subjects and to cover the whole concept of human biology in the pre-clinical stage, possibly leading to a medical science degree after three years. Four broad modules covering (1) medicine and surgery, (2) psychiatry, (3) obstetrics, gynaecology and paediatrics, and (4) community medicine and general practice should constitute the clinical stage, but the qualifying doctor should not be expected to be fully trained. Subsequently the programme for postgraduate training should be systematically planned to give wide-ranging experience in carefully allotted posts, for both hospital specialists and general practitioners, through the development of postgraduate training centres in the district general hospitals. The report also suggested that the number of places in medical schools should be doubled by 1990, that the twelve London schools be merged into six expanded schools and the postgraduate schools consolidated with them, closer links being forged all over the country between the medical schools and multi-faculty universities.

Following the Todd recommendations three new provincial medical schools — Southampton, Nottingham and Leicester — were set up but little progress has been made with the amalgamation of London medical schools. The suggestion regarding medical school numbers has been challenged following the scare that there might be too many doctors to allow satisfactory career progression. By 1983 the BMA argued that medical school intake should be held at the 1979 level and even that assumed a considerable increase in the number of GPs consequent on a reduction of list sizes to an average of 1700.

The philosophy of the Todd report has had an influence throughout medical education, and undergraduate curricula are changing quite substantially.[6] Central Councils for Postgraduate Medical Education exist for England and Wales, Scotland and Northern Ireland, with responsibility for monitoring standards and advising the Regional Postgraduate Committees. Joint Higher Training Committees have now been set up for a number of specialties, to define the scope of special education within the specialties, to establish criteria for posts and inspect them, to recommend patterns of appointments and to provide accreditation. There is, similarly, a Postgraduate Training Committee for General Practice. In 1976 the National Health Service (Vocational Training) Act was passed, creating a legal framework for the future regulation of training for doctors wishing to become general practitioners. Since January 1982 all intending GPs have to take an accredited three-year vocational training course which involves two further years in hospital medicine in appropriate specialties such as obstetrics, geriatrics, paediatrics, psychiatry and general medicine, and one year as a trainee attached to a GP practice.

The Distribution of Hospital Doctors

Career progression in hospital is still a problem. As the DHSS *Medical Manpower*[7] paper pointed out in 1978, the hospital medical staffing structure is an 'uneasy pyramidal shape' maintained largely by the employment of overseas doctors and by using junior doctors as 'pairs of hands' rather than as trainees. The Todd report had suggested an increase in training posts between the registrar and consultant grades. This was rejected by the Royal Commission who suggested a possible solution whereby there would be three grades after registration: an assistant physician (or surgeon), a grade with a tenure of about four years, a physician grade which could be either a final post or act as a training post for the consultant grade. This proposal was not accepted and neither was the suggestion in the King's Fund Study *The Organisation of Hospital Clinical Work*[8] a year later, that there should be two grades of consultant which, it was said, would encourage mobility and allow consultants to change their interests. At present they may hold the same contract for thirty years.

But before discussing the problem of hospital doctors' careers further and in particular the recommendations of the House of Commons Social Services Committee (the Short report)[9] made in July 1981, it is worth being reminded of the present system.

The organisation of hospital doctors in the NHS was first set out by the Spens Committee on the remuneration of consultants and specialists, in 1948,[10] but there have been a number of modifications since that time, notably as a result of the recommendations of the Joint Working Party on Medical Staffing Structure in the Hospital Service (the Platt report[11]) in 1961. The present position is that following registration a young hospital doctor can expect to spend at least one year as a senior house officer, followed by one to three years as a registrar and three to five years as a senior registrar before becoming a consultant in his late thirties. However, the actual position varies a great deal and orderly progression is not ensured since there are many more aspiring junior doctors than there are consultant posts which they stand a chance of obtaining. Some of the junior (i.e. non-consultant) posts are regarded as service rather than training posts, implying that the manpower is needed to fulfil a hospital's clinical obligations and not to provide training and experience which will entitle the holder to automatic promotion.

The clinical work is organised around a basic unit called a 'firm', composed of one consultant and a varying number from the junior grades. Patients referred to hospital by a GP for inpatient or outpatient treatment become the responsibility of the consultant, who has to make decisions about their diagnosis, treatment, referral and discharge. He is helped by his junior doctors and by a variety of nursing and paramedical staff, and delegates some of the work to them while retaining full personal responsibility. In practice the senior registrars and registrars have some autonomy although they are responsible to their consultant, and they supervise the work of the house officers. The discretion given to each grade of junior doctor varies considerably from 'firm' to 'firm', and depends on the nature of the clinical work, the number of staff involved and the inevitable personality influences. Teaching of junior medical staff, medical students and other hospital staff may also play a part in the work of the 'firm'.

At the next level, clinical work done by the 'firms' is organised into specialties (see Figure 23). Figures from the DHSS show that some specialties are much more popular than others, and the competition in some is so severe that a trainee is not assured a career post in

Figure 24 *Hospital Consultants Distinction Awards.* Distinction award holders in England and Wales at 31 December 1982: analysis of type of award, specialty, and percentage distribution

Specialty	Eligible practitioners		Award holders										Non-award holders	
			Total		A+		A		B		C			
	No	%	No	%	No	%	No	%	No	%	No	%	No	%
All specialties: Total	14,191	100	5,068	35.7	125	0.9	462	3.3	1,357	9.6	3,124	22.0	9,123	64.3
Anaesthetics	1,710	12.0	489	28.6	12	0.7	25	1.5	107	6.3	345	20.2	1,221	71.4
Cardiology	126	0.9	71	56.3	5	4.0	12	9.5	27	21.4	27	21.4	55	43.7
Cardio-thoracic surgery	111	0.8	65	58.6	1	0.9	17	15.3	22	19.8	25	22.5	46	41.4
Clinical neurological physiology	46	0.3	13	28.3	—	—	—	—	7	15.2	6	13.0	33	71.7
Community medicine	558	3.9	135	24.2	1	0.2	16	2.9	30	5.4	88	15.8	423	75.8
Dental surgery	305	2.2	119	39.0	4	1.3	8	2.6	39	12.8	68	22.3	186	61.0
Orthodontics	133	0.9	42	31.6	1	0.8	4	3.0	9	6.8	28	21.0	91	68.4
Restorative dentistry	79	0.6	21	26.6	—	—	3	3.8	3	3.8	15	19.0	58	73.4
Dermatology	213	1.5	81	38.0	1	0.5	10	4.7	22	10.3	48	22.5	132	62.0
Diseases of the chest	167	1.2	77	46.1	1	0.6	5	3.0	21	12.6	50	29.9	90	53.9
Ear, nose and throat	379	2.7	134	35.4	2	0.5	7	1.8	35	9.2	90	23.7	245	64.6
General medicine	1,324	9.3	598	45.2	24	1.8	74	5.6	167	12.6	333	25.2	726	54.8
General surgery	1,102	7.8	546	49.6	15	1.4	53	4.8	158	14.3	320	29.0	556	50.4
Genito-urinary medicine	110	0.8	22	20.0	—	—	3	2.7	9	8.2	10	9.1	88	80.0
Geriatric medicine	426	3.0	104	24.4	4	0.9	5	1.2	23	5.4	72	16.9	322	75.6
Infectious diseases	28	0.2	15	53.6	1	3.6	2	7.1	3	10.7	9	32.1	13	46.4
Mental illness	1,124	7.9	322	29.5	10	0.9	19	1.7	81	7.2	222	19.7	792	70.5
Child and adolescent psychiatry	336	2.4	68	20.2	1	0.3	5	1.5	19	5.7	43	12.8	268	79.8
Forensic psychiatry	25	0.2	7	28.0	—	—	1	4.0	—	—	6	24.0	18	72.0
Mental handicap	153	1.1	36	23.5	—	—	4	2.6	5	3.3	27	17.6	117	76.5
Psychotherapy	74	0.5	14	18.9	—	—	—	—	5	6.8	9	12.2	60	81.1

Figure 24 (contd)

Neurology	156	1.1	78	50.0	2	1.3	7	4.5	24	15.4	45	28.9	78	50.0
Neurosurgery	96	0.7	55	57.3	1	1.0	12	12.5	18	18.8	24	25.0	41	42.7
Nuclear medicine	24	0.2	15	62.5		–	1	4.2	5	20.8	9	37.5	9	37.5
Obstetrics and gynaecology	714	5.0	275	38.5	10	1.4	27	3.8	67	9.4	171	23.9	439	61.5
Ophthalmology	407	2.9	142	34.9	1	0.2	10	2.5	39	9.6	92	22.6	265	65.1
Orthopaedic surgery	681	4.8	225	33.0	2	0.3	14	2.1	53	7.8	156	22.9	456	67.0
Accident and Emergency	125	0.9	17	13.6	–	–	–	–	1	0.8	16	12.8	108	86.4
Paediatrics	548	3.9	202	36.9	7	1.3	12	2.2	57	10.4	126	23.0	346	63.1
Paediatric surgery	39	0.3	25	64.1	2	5.1	4	10.3	4	10.3	15	38.5	14	35.9
Pathology – general	8	0.1	3	37.5	–	–	–	–	1	12.5	2	25.0	5	62.5
Blood tranfusion	34	0.2	12	35.3	–	–	1	3.0	2	5.9	9	26.5	22	64.7
Chemical pathology	173	1.2	82	47.4	1	0.6	12	6.9	24	13.9	45	26.0	91	52.6
Haematology	357	2.5	108	30.3	1	0.3	11	3.1	27	7.6	69	19.3	249	69.7
Histopathology	530	3.7	206	38.9	2	0.4	26	4.9	54	10.2	124	23.4	324	61.1
Immuno-pathology	42	0.3	14	33.3	–	–	–	2.4	7	16.7	6	14.3	28	66.7
Medical microbiology	298	2.1	108	36.2	1	0.3	7	2.3	30	10.1	70	23.5	190	63.8
Neuropathology	33	0.2	18	54.5	1	3.0	3	9.1	9	27.3	5	15.2	15	45.5
PHLS only	39	0.3	16	41.0	–	–	1	2.6	4	10.3	11	28.2	23	59.0
Plastic surgery	87	0.6	38	43.7	–	1.2	4	4.6	12	13.8	21	24.1	49	56.3
Radiology	847	6.0	276	32.6	6	0.7	19	2.2	73	8.6	178	21.0	571	67.4
Radiotherapy	199	1.4	89	44.7	3	1.5	9	4.5	38	19.1	39	19.6	110	55.3
Rheumatology and rehabilitation	225	1.6	75	33.3	1	0.4	8	3.6	16	7.1	50	22.2	150	66.7

Source: DHSS, *Health Trends*, vol. 15, p. 67, August 1983, London

any of the following specialties: clinical physiology, nephrology, cardiology, infectious diseases, general surgery, obstetrics and gynaecology, ophthalmology, urology, neurosurgery and paediatric surgery. On the other hand, registrars specialising in geriatrics, venereology, chemical pathology and anaesthetics can be sure of obtaining senior registrar posts; and all senior registrars in these same four specialties plus child psychiatry and radiology can expect to obtain a consultant post on completion of their training.

The Short report endeavoured to deal with the problems which had been troubling the NHS for some years. It recommended increasing the number of consultants and improving the training of hospital doctors aspiring to be consultants. The report recognised that despite the relatively large number of junior doctors it was not always easy to find good candidates for certain consultant posts. However, it did not accept that more junior posts were the answer to this problem, despite the overlong hours that many junior doctors worked. The solution offered was a substantial increase in the number of consultants to ensure a consultant based service which would increase the benefits to patients many of whom at present only saw a consultant very briefly. To encourage an increase in consultants, the number of senior house officer posts should be frozen at the 1981 level. Somewhat surprisingly these proposals were not received well by consultants, although they were welcomed by the junior staff. The consultants were offended at the implication that many of them had little knowledge of their patients and they were doubtful whether the career progression could be so finely tuned; in other words, some wastage during training was not only inevitable, but possibly desirable to ensure that only the most suitable doctors became consultants. In any case, it takes time and experience for doctors to decide on a specialty. A recent study showed that on qualifying only a quarter of doctors had made up their minds about career preference.[12] In subsequent discussions, it became clear that a reduction in juniors' working hours in smaller specialties would mean the consultants themselves being first on-call on some occasions — and this was felt to be unacceptable.

Previous reports on medical matters have been criticised initially only to be found acceptable later on. Presumably working on this premise, the DHSS issued a circular early in 1982, HC(82)4, which accompanied the government's response to the Short report and welcomed and supported most of the report's recommendations. In particular, RHAs were asked to prevent further expansion of senior house officer posts and to draw up plans aimed at achieving by 1988 a ratio of 1:1 of consultants to training grade posts and to evaluate the cost of this. Progress has been slow. The freeze on senior house officers has been implemented, but its effects have been arbitrary leaving imbalances in the number of these posts between specialties. The Short report had suggested that junior medical staff contracts should be held at the Region, to facilitate the redeployment of posts. This change has not been made and neither has the corresponding proposal, strongly supported in paragraph 21 of *Patients First*, that consultants' contracts should be held by DHAs rather than RHAs. Individual health authorities have been encouraged by the DHSS and Regions to increase the number of consultant posts, particularly in the less popular specialties, but such posts have to be funded from within the allocation and money has not always been available. In September 1982, for instance, there were 635 vacant consultant posts which were not even being advertised.

Two other problems connected with the distribution of hospital doctors are the role of overseas doctors and the need to retrain or retain women doctors. Both these groups tend to have an unpredictable effect on manpower plans. The Royal Commission estimated that of the 18,000 UK registered doctors who had been born outside the UK and Eire, half had come from the Indian sub-continent and a quarter from Australia, Canada and New Zealand. It was estimated (1979) that about a fifth of the number entered and left the NHS each year.[13] The GMC's introduction of more stringent language and accreditation procedures was expected to reduce the number of overseas doctors, but a proportion wish to stay in the NHS and to become consultants. Early in 1984 the Secretary of State was approached by the BMA to reduce the number of overseas doctors even further. This move was deplored by the Overseas Doctors Association. As in most professions, women doctors have had more difficulty in planning their careers than men. The Royal Commission estimated that 70 per cent of trained women doctors worked in medicine in some capacity, but this was compared with over 90 per cent of male doctors. Attempts have been made through the Women Doctors Retainer Scheme introduced in 1972,[14] to enable previously unemployed women doctors to undertake part-time work to keep in touch with their profession. The retraining scheme[15] inaugurated in 1969 makes special arrangements for women to work part-time at registrar and senior registrar level. Inevitably, women do better in shortage specialties and in those specialties such as community medicine where there are permanent sub-consultant grade posts.

General Practitioners

The split between general practitioners and hospital doctors that emerged in the 18th and 19th centuries still exists, and general practice, although it has in the lifetime of the NHS consistently attracted about 50 per cent of qualifying doctors, remains the less prestigious choice. Both the Royal College of General Practitioners and the General Medical Services Committee (GMSC) of the BMA have worked hard to improve the standing of general practice and there is a growing recognition of the fact that general practice as the key element of primary medical care is the area where more planning of services and scrutiny of the outcome of treatment will be able to alter the balance in the whole pattern of health care. The GMSC issued a booklet late in 1983[16] reviewing the present state of general practice. It concluded that general practice remained a stable and widely appreciated part of the NHS providing the bulk of health care, and there was room for further development, particularly in reducing list size to allow doctors to spend more time with their patients. Between 1949 and 1978 the number of GPs increased by 36 per cent compared with an increase of hospital doctors of well over 100 per cent. This increase in GPs has allowed the average list size to decrease so that in 1981 there were 27,484 GP principals with an average list size of 2,146. As has already been stated it is the aim of the BMA to reduce the list size to 1,700 although there are some doctors who feel that with appropriate organisation GPs could see more patients rather than less. Within these figures there are important local variations. In order to secure an even distribution of GPs throughout the country the National Health Service Act 1946 established a 9 member independent body called the Medical Practices Committee (MPC) who were made responsible for controlling the number of GPs operating in any one area. They did this by introducing four categories; *designated areas* – with an average list of over 2,500; *open areas* – between 2,101 and 2,500; *intermediate areas* – between 1,701 and 2,100; *restricted areas* – 1,700 or less. Doctors wishing to practice have to apply to the FPC for approval but in the case of a restricted area the MPC cannot recommend approval. Correspondingly, financial inducements are offered to those wishing to practice in designated areas. Family Practitioner Committees are responsible for reporting vacancies to the MPC and making recommendations regarding the filling of posts which will take into account population changes and other developments. FPCs fill the vacancies once they have been authorised by the MPC and hold the GPs' contracts.

General practitioners' remuneration is made up of several elements. Figure 25 shows where GPs have opportunities to increase their earnings

Figure 25 *General Practitioners' Pay*

	Present fees and allowances (£)	Review body's recommen- dations (£)	OME's recalculated rates (£)
Full rate of basic practice allowance	5755	6030	5935
Additions to basic practice allowance:			
Designated area allowance:			
Type I	1795	1880	1850
Type II	2735	2865	2820
Group practice allowance	1005	1055	1035
Seniority allowance:			
First stage	1385	1450	1430
Second stage	2360	2475	2435
Third stage	3740	3920	3860
Vocational training allowance	1385	1450	1430
Standard capitation fees:			
Patients under 65	5.30	5.65	5.55
Patients aged 65 to 74	6.85	7.35	7.20
Patients aged 75 and over	8.45	9.00	8.85
Payments for out of hours responsibilities:			
Supplementary practice allowance (full rate)	1135	1190	1170
Supplementary capitation fee	1.08	1.15	1.13
Night visit fee	12.75	13.35	13.15
Item of service fees:			
Vaccination and immunisation:			
Lower rate	1.90	2.00	1.95
Higher rate	2.70	2.85	2.80
Cervical cytology test	5.40	5.70	5.60
Contraceptive service fees:			
Ordinary fee	7.30	7.65	7.55
Intrauterine dervice fee	24.55	25.75	25.30
Maternity services fee (doctors on obstetric list)	77.65	88.25	86.75
Temporary resident fees:			
Patients expecting to remain in the district for:			
Not more than 15 days	4.20	4.40	4.35
More than 15 days	6.35	6.60	6.55
Fees for emergency treatment:			
Minor surgical operation involving local or general anaesthetic	10.90	11.40	11.25
Administration of any other general anaesthetic	18.25	19.15	18.80
Postgraduate training allowance	520	545	535
Training grant under trainee practitioner scheme	3105	3160	3160
Rural practice funds		+ 4.8%	+ 3.1%
Average remuneration from on cost and professional fees per unrestricted principal in respect of dispensing and supply of drugs and appliances		+ 4.8%	+ 3.1%

Source: Calculations by Office of Manpower Economics based on the Thirteenth Report of the Review Body on Doctors' and Dentists' Remuneration, 1983.

if they so wish. In addition, they can apply to become clinical assistants or hospital practitioners helping consultants in hospital work. The number of GPs working alone has steadily fallen and most doctors now work in a partnership of three or more, well supported by staff such as receptionists and secretaries. District nurses, health visitors and occasionally health workers attached to the practice have developed the team approach, particularly important in family medicine.

Patients are generally satisfied with access to their doctors, but concern regarding deputising arrangements, particularly in inner-city areas, led to government proposals in 1983 to eliminate the use of deputies in large practices and restrict their use for GPs working alone. It was estimated that if regulations were introduced only a fifth of GPs would still be allowed to use deputising services. As the services are often provided by junior hospital medical staff, they would stand to lose valuable extra income.

Doctors and Management

The participation of hospital doctors in management and their contribution to the efficiency of the hospital service was a major theme of the first reorganisation and stemmed from the fact that doctors were in a position to direct the use of costly resources with varying, but often considerable, degrees of autonomy. After discussions between the Minister of Health and the profession in 1965, the Joint Working Party on the Organisation of Medical Work in Hospitals was set up to discuss the progress of the NHS and particularly to review the hospital service. It produced three reports (1967,[17] 1972,[18] 1974[19]) known as the Cogwheel reports because of the design printed on their covers. The first report recommended the creation of divisions of broadly linked specialties to include consultants and junior medical staff which would constantly appraise their services and methods of provision. Such divisions were likely to be set up on a faculty or specialty basis, such as surgery, medicine, obstetrics, pathology, etc. Representatives of each division were to come together in each hospital as a medical executive committee which would coordinate the work and views of the division and provide a link with nursing and administration. The sort of problems they might consider included bed management and the organisation of outpatient and inpatient resources. Most hospital groups gradually implemented this scheme, and by 1972 the second report was able to identify the essential elements of an effective Cogwheel system and to report that in large acute hospitals particularly, the system had been helpful in dealing with improved communications, reductions of inpatient waiting lists and the progressive control of medical expenditure.

The third report clarified the role of Cogwheel systems in the newly reorganised NHS, because an emphasis of the 1974 reorganisation was the part to be played by multidisciplinary teams in the integrated management, whereas Cogwheel had been set up as a doctor dominated hospital based arrangement. The third report suggested that Cogwheel should continue to deal with issues where the agreement and action of hospital doctors was the main need, while problems requiring strong collaboration between all the professional groups, both within the hospitals and in community services should be the province of the district management teams and their health care planning teams. It would still be appropriate for Cogwheel systems to concentrate on efficiency issues, and it would be helpful for hospital doctors to see their clinical freedom in the context of team work and the necessity of sharing resources.

Cogwheel divisions have not flourished everywhere, however, but where they have many have required a considerable amount of administrative support. Support for the Cogwheel concept is nevertheless fairly general, if at times somewhat grudging; certainly an alternative is difficult to find given the clinical autonomy which consultants claim and largely have. The Royal Commission noted an impatience amongst medical staff with the seemingly inevitable delays intrinsic within consensus management and they supported an executive team at hospital level which they thought would speed things up. The idea of unit management teams was endorsed in *Patients First* and in circular HC(80)8[20] on the new structure, but the involvement of doctors was somewhat ambiguously stated. It was not until HC(82)1[21] that clear directions were given on how clinical members were to be appointed to the DMT following the 1982 reorganisation. The consultant should be elected by the consultant body and the GP by all GPs in a District. This marked a change in some places where previously the District Medical Committee, itself a representative body, had elected the DMT medical representatives. These representatives usually serve for a limited period.

Following the 1982 reorganisation, unit management teams were set up usually as a triumvirate of doctor, nurse and administrator, but in some cases included hospital doctors and GPs. The role of these teams has not been altogether easy to determine, and nor has their corporate relationship to the DMT. The 1983 Griffiths report proposals recommended modification to this type of team decision making. Ironically, it was hospital doctors' criticisms of consensus management which probably did most to encourage the Secretary of State to ask for the Griffiths report in the first place. The resulting proposals that there should be a general manager at District and Unit level led the BMA to say that such a post should be held by a doctor, even though many doctors were doubtful that filling the role would be practicable given their comparative or total lack of management training and their prime commitment to patient treatment which would allow little time for the managerial role.

The dilemma cannot be easily resolved. Doctors need to be involved closely in the decisions about health care, but cannot spend too much time away from their patients. It remains to be seen whether the Griffiths proposals are an effective improvement on Cogwheel and on consensus management.

To a certain extent the idea of a top doctor had been tried before with the medical superintendent in some hospitals and with the Medical Officer of Health in local health authorities prior to the 1974 reorganisation. Medical superintendents' posts atrophied well before 1974, but the Medical Officer of Health was a highly influential officer in local authorities whose work was widely appreciated. The holders of these posts did not find it altogether easy to adapt to the different management principles following that reorganisation and this has left community medicine in a somewhat ambiguous position. Possibly this is one of the reasons there are relatively few community physicians (815 in September 1982). Is community medicine about the management of medical work or is it about the management of the community's health? Despite the claims of the Hunter report (*Report of the Working Party on Medical Administrators* (1972))[22] which had tried to amalgamate both the managerial and clinical responsibilities, the Royal Commission felt that the community physicians' role in planning, health education, epidemiology and environmental control should be encouraged. This implied that the more administrative tasks should be undertaken by administrators.

Doctors' Pay

Doctors' pay has often been a significant problem for governments to handle. Doctors' negotiators have been no less dedicated than other groups of workers and industrial action has not been unknown. In order to understand the present position, it helps to give a brief account of the history of doctors' pay negotiations.

When the NHS began, the systems for employing the services of doctors had had to be carefully worked out and negotiated between the government and the profession. Two committees under the chairmanship of Sir Will Spens reported in 1948 on the remuneration of general practitioners,[23] and consultants and specialists respectively. They recommended scales for consultants and junior hospital doctors, arrangements for part-time contracts for consultants and a system of distinction awards which would provide for a significant minority the opportunity to earn incomes comparable with the highest which can be earned in other professions.[24] For GPs the Spens committee recommended a graded scale of incomes leading to an average net income for doctors of forty to fifty years of age, which would be paid out of a central pool. The GPs' income would be made up of a capitation fee for each patient on his list, which included a fixed allowance for practice expenses, plus payments for certain individual items of service. The figures for all doctors were quoted at 1939 values of money, it being left for the government to decide what increases would establish and protect the status of these incomes relative to each other and to other professional incomes, in the context of rising inflation.

The adjustments that were accordingly fixed by the government were not acceptable to the BMA in respect of GPs' incomes, and after negotiations had broken down, the matter was referred to adjudication in 1953. Mr Justice Danckwerts awarded the GPs a substantial increase and said that the size of the central pool should be related to the total number of GPs and not to the population covered by the NHS, in order that required increases in the numbers of GPs would not be discouraged. The result was that some of the increased incomes were paid directly into a special fund from which GPs could draw if they spent money on improving or building new surgery premises.

The BMA again made a claim for increases in 1956, but this time on behalf of hospital doctors as well as GPs. The Health Ministers could not agree to it and the matter was referred to a Royal Commission under Sir Harry Pilkington, which sat from 1957 to 1960.[25] It recommended new levels of remuneration but also that a standing review body of '. . . eminent persons of experience in various fields of national life'[26] should keep medical and dental remuneration under review, making recommendations directly to the Prime Minister, which were on the whole to be accepted without alteration. The BMA refused to give evidence to the Royal Commission, but when the Presidents of the Royal Colleges announced that they would cooperate by putting the view of hospital consultants and specialists, the BMA was left with no alternative if it wished the GPs to have a voice but to submit a brief to the Commission. The effect of setting up a review body was to end the practice initiated by Spens of calculating doctors' pay increases in relation to the rate of inflation, but at the same time it left the pay settlements in the hands of a body separate from the Ministry that could be advised but not instructed by the government. Chapter 11 will describe how the Whitley Council system for collective bargaining and determination of the pay of all NHS staff was set up and how it has operated. In the case of doctors, the Royal Commission was persuaded to recommend the end of direct negotiations between representatives of the health departments and the profession on Whitley Councils through the creation of a permanent independent review body.

The Review Body on Doctors' and Dentists' Remuneration was duly set up, consisting of six members and the Chairman, Lord Kindersley. Its terms of reference were 'to advise the Prime Minister on the remuneration of doctors and dentists taking any part in the National Health Service'. Twelve reports were issued between 1963 and 1970 and these concerned the basic rates of pay for different grades of doctors and dentists as well as particular aspects of remuneration including distinction awards. The review body constructed its recommendations after receiving evidence from doctors' and dentists' representatives, from the Ministry/DHSS, and factual information about changes in the cost of living, the movement of earnings in other professions and the state of recruitment in the profession. However, general practitioners were not satisfied with the awards made to them by the review body, and in 1965 the BMA submitted a memorandum demanding direct reimbursement of practice expenses and of income from local authority and hospital sessional work, a system of seniority payments and a number of other items. The review body made an award of £5½ million, on the condition that most of it would be used to reimburse those doctors employing ancillary help or spending above-average amounts in improving their services for patients. The BMA replied (through its General Medical Services Committee) that this award and previous awards which maintained the pool system could not enable GPs to secure 'just' remuneration. They demanded an immediate unconditional credit of the £5½ million award to the

pool — thus raising the value of the capitation fee — as an interim
measure, and asked GPs throughout the country to sign undated
resignation forms which would be used or not, depending on the outcome of negotiations with the Minister.[27] In March 1965, Kenneth
Robinson (the Minister of Health since October 1964) agreed to add
the £5½ million unconditionally to the pool, and began discussing the
GPs' suggestion for a completely new contract, as outlined in the
BMA's publication *A Charter for the Family Doctor Service*.[28] This set
out a radically revised scheme of payments, including a 5½-day working
week, six weeks paid annual holiday, payments for out-of-hours
services, an independent corporation to make long-term loans to GPs
for building or improving surgery premises, the ending of the pool
system, direct reimbursement for practice expenses, ancillary help,
and several other items. Long negotiations on the Charter ensued and
a contract jointly agreed to by the Minister and the profession which
embodied some but not all of the demands was submitted to the review
body for pricing, later in 1965. It consisted of a basic payment, available at the full rate to doctors with at least 1,000 patients providing
full services for a minimum period in each week, and available to other
doctors at proportionally reduced rates. Additions to this were made
in respect of group practice and practice in unattractive areas. Two
levels of distinction awards were available to about 30 per cent of GPs
aged between forty-five and sixty-five, depending on attendance at a
required number of postgraduate training courses. Additional services
provided by GPs in accordance with national policy, e.g. cervical
cytology and vaccination and immunisation, were to be paid on an
item-of-service basis, as were maternity and emergency work. The
capitation fees for ordinary weekday work were fixed at two rates,
that for patients over sixty-five being about 30 per cent higher than for
other patients. Night-time and weekend work earned the GP an
additional standby allowance, and extra capitation fee for over 1,000
patients, and a flat rate for home visits made between midnight and
7.00 a.m. Six weeks paid annual holiday plus a notional 5½-day week
were established, provided that the GP could make arrangements for
the complete care of his patients while he was not working. The BMA's
Charter would have cost an extra £38 million, but the review body's
recommendations on the jointly agreed package resulted in an extra
cost of about £24 million to the NHS. Although the GPs did not get
exactly what they had demanded, the gap between the incomes of GPs
and hospital consultants was narrowed. A notable achievement of the
whole dispute was, however, to encourage group practice from purpose

built or modified premises, through the setting up of the General Practice Finance Corporation, and the reimbursement of a greater proportion of practice expenses which encouraged employment of ancillary staff. It also reduced the burden of signing National Insurance certificates, which the GPs strongly objected to.

In March 1970 the twelfth report of the review body[29] recommended a general increase of 30 per cent for doctors and dentists to be introduced over two years, because their pay had been falling behind increases for other professions. The government accepted this for the training grades of doctors and dentists but only agreed to half the awards for career grades in hospital and general practice work, referring the balance to the National Board for Prices and Incomes. In June, Lord Kindersley and the members of the Review Board resigned on the day after this announcement, and the BMA advised its members not to cooperate with the NHS administration. These sanctions were lifted after the general election in 1970 in return for assurances from the new Conservative government that the reference to the National Board for Prices and Incomes would be withdrawn. In November 1970 the government set up three new review bodies to handle the pay negotiations for groups in the public sector where the negotiating machinery had been unsatisfactory — namely, doctors and dentists in the NHS, the chairman and board members of the nationalised industries and the armed forces. These review bodies have interlocking membership and their secretariat is provided from the Office of Manpower Economics. The new terms of reference for the doctors' and dentists' review body (chaired by Lord Halsbury) laid down that their recommendations would not be referred to another body (this had been the reason for Lord Kindersley's resignation) and would not be rejected or modified unless it was unavoidable.

Lord Halsbury resigned as Chairman of the review body after the fourth report,[30] published in July 1974, had been rejected by the profession who expressed their lack of confidence in him. The review body continued its work without a chairman, and published a supplement[31] to the fourth report at the end of the year. This was accepted by the government and the profession. Annual reports have been issued since then.

For hospital doctors, relations with the government were not so troublesome until about 1972 when dissatisfactions with the form of consultants' contracts arose. The consultants' view, expressed mainly through the BMA, was that they had been required to take on several new responsibilities without adequate pay adjustments. At that time their contracts specified the minimum number of hours to be worked, depending on whether the doctor had opted to work whole-time for the NHS, or part-time in order to take on private work also. The system of distinction awards also made extra annual payments of between £1,500 and £8,000 (approximately) to a proportion of consultants. Discussions between the consultants and the Department continued inconclusively, and in 1974 a general election replaced the Conservatives with a Labour government. The new Secretary of State for Social Services, Mrs Barbara Castle, took up the consultants' problem by proposing to make full-time NHS work more financially attractive than part-time work. In addition she proposed to recast the distinction awards system entirely by creating two new pay supplements: a medical progress supplement (to award valuable innovations in medical research or academic study, like the old awards) and a service supplement (to reward overburdened consultants in unpopular regions or unfashionable specialties, which the old awards neglected). Negotiations on these proposals were stormy, and took place in the context of the review body's deliberations on a claim from the consultants for a large interim backdated increase. At the beginning of 1975 the BMA called on consultants to 'work to contract' – i.e. to do no more than the minimum they were required to do – to demonstrate their opposition to the government's proposals and their rejection of the review body's decision not to grant them an interim award. The disruption caused by the consultants' action was quite widespread, but it ceased later in 1975.

At about the same time, however, junior hospital doctors commenced to 'work to contract' in support of their claims for a new contract to recognise the long hours and heavy responsibilities they had to shoulder. Again, the negotiations were acrimonious but a settlement was reached later in 1975 when the review body priced two new types of supplement that junior doctors could receive if they worked extra hours over a newly defined basic working week of 40 hours. The cost of this settlement turned out to be more expensive than the review body had calculated, because of the way the health authorities awarded the new supplements. In addition, hospital work levels were significantly reduced as a result of the consultants' and junior doctors' 'working to contract', and this showed up as increased waiting times for outpatient appointments and inpatient admissions.

The junior doctors' new contract took effect from February 1976, but despite extensive discussion a new contract for consultants has not materialised. No further progress on changing the system of distinction awards has been made. The tasks of the review body, in the light of these disputes and under the constraints imposed by the government's pay policy, has been made extremely difficult. The review body was after all set up to avoid recurrent disputes and to arrive at settlements which would be fair to the profession and to the taxpayer who foots the bill. In the event, the effect of increasing militancy amongst members of the medical profession, and government attempts to control the rate of pay increases, has put great strains on the ability of both sides to negotiate acceptable pay and terms of work under the NHS. As an indication of their frustration, the junior doctors decided in 1978 to ask the DHSS to negotiate directly with them about pay, instead of relying on the review body. However, the junior doctors did not get their way and the BMA's Review Body Evidence Committee is now made up of representatives of not only the hospital junior staff committee (HJSC) but also the Central Committee for Hospital and Medical Services (CCHMS), the General Medical Services Committee (GMSC), the Central Committee for Community Medicine (CCCM) and a single representative of the Ophthalmic Group Committee (OGC).

Intrinsic problems persist with the negotiation of doctors' pay. The review body when first set up seemed to be more sensitive and more influential than the Whitley Council, but it has also been politically more vulnerable to governments who can negotiate settlements on the assumption that doctors will not get any support from other groups of staff and their trade unions. As has been seen, the professional representatives of the review body are not always in accord and at least twice in the last ten years the junior medical staff have had serious disagreements with their parent body, the BMA. Another problem with pay is that of relativities. Doctors have been able to demonstrate from time to time that they have done less well over time than other groups of staff. But in 1983, prior to the general election, they received a two year agreement which was significantly better than that received by other health workers. Fairness is very difficult to establish, but whatever the variations over a period, doctors seem able to remain the best paid group of health care staff overall. This is partly because their contracts have advantageous elements not available to others. Many consultants can do private work in addition to their NHS contract. Since 1979 even full consultants are allowed to earn up to 10 per cent of their full-time salary in private medicine. Domiciliary visit fees (approximately £22.00 per visit) can be claimed with a normal top limit of 300 visits per year. Distinction awards are held by 36 per cent of hospital doctors (see Figure 23). For junior medical staff a type of overtime payment now increases their basic income by over 36 per cent. These units of medical time (UMTs), the fruits of the 1975 dispute, were originally meant to distinguish between time standing-by in the hospital ('A' UMTs) and time on-call at home ('B' UMTs). In practice 'B' UMTs are seldom allocated. The problem of long hours remains; a junior doctor works an average of 84 hours a week, but it should be noted that 44 per cent of that time on average is spent in the hospital available for work rather than being in actual contact with patients. Some specialties are better staffed than others and negotiations since the Short report have endeavoured to ensure that no junior doctor has to work on a more than 1 in 3 night rota.[32] As this may involve providing cover to a specialty other than their own, it has yet to be achieved and indeed agreed by juniors and their consultants.

The Royal Commission was uneasy with the junior doctors' style of contract which in its view moved away from the traditional role of the doctor who assumed total care of his patients regardless of time. The work-sensitive contract of the juniors was seen as an unhappy departure from the traditions of British medicine. The trouble was, however, that such traditions undoubtedly exploited junior medical staff. The alternative, which looks increasingly like a shift system, would, however, sacrifice continuity of care for the patient and would require more administration to support the handover from one shift to the next.

Notes

1. Further Medical Acts, passed in 1956 and 1969, consolidated amendments to the membership and powers of the Council.

2. *Report of the Committee of Enquiry into the Regulations of the Medical Profession* (Chairman, Dr A.W. Merrison), HMSO, London, 1975 (Cmnd. 6018). The GMC had decided to change the registration system to require doctors to pay an annual fee instead of the existing once-only payment. Doctors refused to comply with this so if the GMC had proceeded with the new system, the NHS would have been forced to employ non-registered doctors – an illegal arrangement. The inquiry into the GMC was announced to forestall the problem, and the committee itself decided to widen its brief to look at medical education and training as well as the membership and activities of the GMC.

3. Ministry of Health. *Report of the Interdepartmental Committee on Medical Schools* (Chairman, Sir William Goodenough), HMSO, London, 1944.

4. *Royal Commission on Medical Education* (Chairman, Lord Todd), HMSO, London, 1968 (Cmnd. 3569).

5. Equivalent qualifications were also issued by the Conjoint Board of the Royal Colleges of Physicians and Surgeons (MRCS, LRCP) and by the Society of Apothecaries (LMSSA).

6. See the GMC's recent survey: *Basic Medical Education in the British Isles*, Nuffield Provincial Hospitals Trust, London, 1978.

7. DHSS. *Medical Manpower – The next twenty years*, HMSO, London, 1978.

8. King's Fund Project Paper No. 22. *The Organisation of Hospital Clinical Work*, King's Fund, London, 1979.

9. House of Commons. Social Services Committee. Session 1980–81. Fourth Report. *Medical Education with Special Reference to the Number of Doctors and the Career Structure in Hospitals*. (Chairman, Renee Short MP).

10. Ministry of Health and Department of Health for Scotland. *Report of the Inter-Departmental Committee on the Remuneration of Consultants and Specialists* (Chairman, Sir Will Spens), HMSO, London, 1948 (Cmnd. 7420).

11. Ministry of Health and Department of Health for Scotland. *Medical Staffing Structure in the Hospital Service: Report of the Joint Working Party* (Chairman, Sir Robert Platt), HMSO, London, 1961.

12. DHSS. *Health Trends*, Vol. 15, No. 2, p. 29, London, May 1983.

13. *Royal Commission on the National Health Service*, para. 14.34, p. 217, HMSO, London, 1979.

14. DHSS. Circular HM(72)42. *Women Doctors' Retainer Scheme*, 1972.

15. DHSS. Circular HM(69)6. *Reemployment of Women Doctors*, 1969.

16. BMA. *General Practice – A British Success*, General Medical Services Committee, London, 1983.

17. Ministry of Health. *First Report of the Joint Working Party on the Organisation of Medical Work in Hospitals*, HMSO, London, 1967.

18. Department of Health and Social Security. *Second Report of the Joint Working Party on the Organisation of Medical Work in Hospitals*, HMSO, London, 1972.

19. Department of Health and Social Security. *Third Report of the Joint Working Party on the Organisation of Medical Work in Hospitals*, HMSO, London, 1974.

20. DHSS Circular HC(80)8. *Health Service Development. Structure and Management*, July 1980.

21. DHSS Circular HC(21)1. *Health Service Development. Professional Advisory Machinery*, January 1982.

22. DHSS. *Report of the Working Party on Medical Administrators* (Chairman, Dr R.B. Hunter), HMSO, London, 1972.

23. Ministry of Health and Department of Health for Scotland. *Report of the Inter-Departmental Committee on the Remuneration of General Practitioners* (Chairman, Sir Will Spens), HMSO, London, 1946.

24. Ibid., p. 10, para. 12.

25. *Royal Commission on Doctors' and Dentists' Remuneration* (Chairman, Sir Harry Pilkington), HSMO, London, 1960 (Cmnd. 939).

26. Ibid., p. 145, para. 428.

27. In fact a total of 17,800 forms were eventually returned.

28. British Medical Association. 'A Charter for the Family Doctor Service', *British Medical Journal*, 18 March 1965, No. 3138, p. 89.

29. Review Body on Doctors' and Dentists' Remuneration. *Twelfth Report* (Chairman, Lord Kindersley), HMSO, London, 1970 (Cmnd. 4352).

30. Review Body on Doctors' and Dentists' Remuneration. *Fourth Report* (Chairman, Lord Halsbury), HMSO, London, 1974 (Cmnd. 5644).

31. Review Body on Doctors' and Dentists' Remuneration. *Supplement to the Fourth Report*, HMSO, London, 1974 (Cmnd. 5849).

32. The DHSS issued several letters and circulars on the subject, PM(83)37, DH(83)33 and in Advance letter dated June 1983 (MO)3/83 health authorities

were warned that the Terms and Conditions of Service for medical and dental staff would prohibit 'regular rota commitments more onerous than one in two from 1 July 1983'. Not all authorities or specialities were able to conform immediately to this rule.

9 NURSING

In an average District, nursing staff salaries absorb some forty per cent of the total budget. It is particularly important therefore that the management of these resources is effective. During the last fifteen years many changes have been introduced aimed at improving the standards and status of nursing. This chapter first undertakes a brief historical review and then describes the present arrangements for nurse training and the maintenance of nursing standards. Finally the role of nurse managers is discussed.

Hospital Nursing

Nursing began as a vocation — a call to a life of devotion through the alleviation of suffering of others — which was associated with the monks and nuns of some religious orders at about the time that hospitals such as St Bartholemew's (1123) and St Thomas's (1215) were founded. The services were given by men and women who were unskilled, but of 'respectable' parentage and generous outlook. However, from the Reformation (sixteenth century) to the nineteenth century, this tradition lapsed, and care given to the sick was haphazard and became associated with the servant classes of the community. Although several of the great voluntary hospitals were founded during this period, there was little or no provision for nursing, and the work was regarded as a sordid duty fit only for 'broken down and drunk old widows'.[1]

After the mid-nineteenth century attitudes began to change, and the idea of nursing as a vocation was revived. In 1840, Elizabeth Fry founded an Institute of Nursing at Guy's Hospital, where women were trained to nurse under Quaker influence. Florence Nightingale (1820–1910) who came from a cultured and influential upper-class family was herself at the heart of these changes. She went to Paris and to Prussia to train as a nurse, with the intention of returning to improve hospital conditions in Britain. However, when the Crimean War broke out, the reports of chaos and suffering amongst the forces urged her to go to the Crimea herself with thirty trained nurses, where she cared for the wounded and was able to improve the medical services substantially.

190

After her return to England, she was regarded as an influential and publicly respected person, and was thus able to found the Nightingale Training School in 1860 at St Thomas's Hospital. The entrants to it were all respectable ladies, and they were trained in the principles and skills of nursing, such as they were at that time. As a result, three grades of trained nurses became established. Sisters were nurses in charge of a ward, who carried out the doctors' orders and trained and worked with probationer nurses. Night superintendents were in charge of the night staff, and deputised for the matron. The matron herself was a gentlewoman (like the others) and responsible to the hospital authorities not only for the employment and training of nurses, but for a variety of housekeeping and administrative arrangements.

Many of the voluntary hospitals adopted this scheme of training and organisation, but the poor law infirmaries, fever hospitals and asylums were much slower to follow. There was no recognised qualification for psychiatric nursing until 1891, when the Royal Medico-Psychological Society started to issue certificates. The issue of registration for nurses provoked a long and complicated struggle, and the medical profession in particular was determined to see that measures to regulate the practice of nursing were improved. Finally in 1919 the Nurses Registration Acts were passed, establishing the General Nursing Council (GNC) as the registering authority. The GNC was made responsible for keeping a register of nurses who had trained in approved institutions and passed examinations after three years of study. After this time, professions other than nursing began to be open to women (e.g. physiotherapy and radiography) and training schools were set up for them in some hospitals, under the direction of the matron, although the medical superintendent or the secretary of the hospital gradually assumed responsibility for some of the other non-nursing activities. Following the Local Government Act (1929)[2] local authorities took charge of the poor law infirmaries and administered them and the maternity homes through their Medical Officers of Health.

The Nurses Act (1943) recognised the need for a less qualified practical nurse and a two-year training leading to enrolment was approved. The 1949 Nurses Act incorporated male nurses into the main part of the Register (they had been on a separate part since 1919), but not until the 1975 Sex Discrimination Act was passed were men allowed to train as midwives. The 1949 Act was important because it also required money to be set aside specifically for nurse training to be administered by nursing training committees.

After the inception of the NHS in 1948 the status of matrons in the former local authority hospitals definitely improved, but with the moves towards grouping hospitals together and administering them as consolidated units, group secretaries and senior medical staff assumed effective control, and the matrons were left with a reduced but more specialised sphere of responsibility, there being no collective voice for the nursing staff at the level of group administration. During the 1950s senior nursing staff gave up housekeeping duties to the general administration.

The Salmon Report

Shortages of trained nurses and this apparent decline in the status of the profession prompted the government to set up a committee in 1963. Its report, known as the Salmon report,[3] noted that the title 'matron' was applied equally to nursing heads of hospitals with ten beds and with 1,000 beds, and that a distinction between their different duties and rights was not made clear. Furthermore, as men were increasingly joining the profession the titles 'matron' and 'sister' had become anachronistic. It also found that the role of nurses as administrators was poorly defined, and that there was confusion over the relative status of general nursing, midwifery, psychiatric nursing and teaching. The report proposed that status should be determined by the kinds of decisions being made and not by the number of beds controlled or the type of patients nursed. Most senior nurses deciding policy were called 'top managers', those programming policy were called 'middle managers', and those controlling the execution of policy were called 'first-line managers'. The report further introduced the terms: section, unit, area and division, to define a nurse's span of control, and named the senior nursing posts accordingly (see Figure 26).

The Minister of Health and the Secretary of State for Scotland accepted these recommendations and it was suggested that sixteen pilot schemes for introducing the new structure should be set up and evaluated over a period of years. Of course the structure outlined needed to be flexible enough to fit in with the differing local circumstances. It is not therefore possible to generalise about the precise structure adopted in each case, but the idea was that the Chief Nursing Officer was responsible for all nursing services and education in the group and was not identified with an individual hospital within it. She was to be accepted as the head of nursing services by the Hospital

Figure 26 *Senior Nursing Staff Organisation*

LEVEL	GRADE	TITLE	SPHERE
Top managers	10	Chief Nursing Officer	Group
Top managers	9	Principal Nursing Officer	Division
Middle managers	8	Senior Nursing Officer	Area
Middle managers	7	Nursing Officer	Unit
First-line managers	6	Charge Nurse/Ward Sister	Section
	5	Staff Nurse	

Source: Report of the Committee on Senior Nursing Staff Structure, HMSO, 1966

Management Committee or Board of Governors, and was to voice nursing opinion at group level. The Principal Nursing Officer (PNO) became responsible to him or her for the management of a division. A division could be planned on an institutional or a functional basis, to cover, for example, general nursing or maternity work or psychiatric nursing, or teaching. The Senior Nursing Officer would be responsible to the PNO for the management of services within an area; this might be the whole of a separate medium-sized hospital or a number of small hospitals. The Nursing Officer was in charge of a unit, that is three to six medical or surgical wards, or for example, a small suite of operating theatres, a specialised unit or an accident and emergency centre. Charge Nurses (male) or Ward Sisters (female) would control an individual section, which could be a ward or an operating theatre.

Community Nursing

Community nurses include home or district nurses, midwives and health visitors. Their work, unlike that of hospital nurses, owes its development to the voluntary organisations of the nineteenth century. Whereas hospital nurses followed doctors' orders in the care of patients, community nurses worked more independently, under the auspices of voluntary organisations. The title 'health visitor' probably first came into use in 1862 when one such body, the Ladies' Sanitary Reform Association of Manchester and Salford, paid staff to visit people in their district, concentrating on cleanliness, helping the sick and advising mothers on the care of their children. In 1875 the Royal Sanitary Institute (now the Royal Society of Health) was founded 'to promote the health of the people' and began to set examinations for sanitary inspectors. In 1892 Florence Nightingale started a course at North

Buckinghamshire Technical College where 'health missionaries' were trained to meet the needs of 'home health-bringing', and the women thus trained were employed by the local council to visit people in need. The Royal Sanitary Institute set examinations for health visitors and school nurses from 1906, and in 1908 the London County Council passed an act specifying that health visitors should hold a certificate from a society approved by the Local Government Board.

By the turn of the century, infant mortality had risen to the rate of 163 per 1,000, and the need for health visitors to advise and instruct mothers on the proper care of their babies was no longer in doubt. Acts passed in 1907 and 1915 requiring births to be registered provided the means of identifying the problem, and health visitors' work concentrated particularly on infant and maternal welfare. From 1925 to 1962 the Royal Sanitary Institute was the body responsible for examining trained health visitors, after which the Council for Training of Health Visitors became the central body for the whole of the UK. This change arose as a consequence of the Jamieson Report[4] which did much to establish the present role of the health visitor. The Council was jointly set up with the Central Council for the Education and Training of Social Workers by an Act of Parliament, with a common chairman. After the Seebohm report was accepted in 1970, the separation took place, and the body became the Council for the Education and Training of Health Visitors (CETHV). It consisted of thirty-one members representing health visitors, nursing education, medicine, educational interests and some others.

Midwives had been recognised from earliest times. In the seventeenth century they were often well-paid and well-respected women, recognised by the bishop. But the rise of the medical profession caused their status to decline, as the richer families employed doctors to deliver their babies. In the nineteenth century the majority of midwives were 'not only untrained and inexperienced, but ignorant, superstitious and of very low character'.[5] However, the Midwives Institute was founded in 1881 by a group of women who wished to improve the standards and status of midwifery. The Midwives Act was passed in 1902 and it established the Central Midwives Board to keep a roll of approved midwives and to ensure adequate training programmes and standards for good practice. The Ministry of Health was created in 1919 and it took on the supervision of the Central Midwives Board.

Midwifery was practised both in hospital and in the community, but staff came essentially from the voluntary organisations. After 1948, the local health authorities were given the statutory duty under the NHS to provide a domiciliary midwifery service and to supervise standards of practice. The hospitals were required to provide sufficient facilities so that every mother could have her baby delivered in hospital if she so wished. Following the recommendations of the Cranbrook report (1959),[6] and the Peel report (1970),[7] increasing numbers of mothers have chosen this option. Problems have therefore arisen for those midwives only working outside hospital in that they have little experience of delivery. In addition small maternity units are being closed in favour of a centralised consultant supervised unit.

District nursing differs from health visiting and midwifery in that it remained a service provided by voluntary organisations for a much longer period, and in the nineteenth century it had not yet become a well-defined occupation. The history of district nursing is closely connected with the benevolence of William Rathbone in Liverpool, and others, such as the Ranyard nurses. The Queen's Institute of District Nursing was founded with money given to Queen Victoria on her Golden and Diamond Jubilees. It accepted for training nurses who had completed the basic training for registration or enrolment. Under the 1946 NHS Act, local health authorities became responsible for organising the home nursing services and they tended to use the established local Queen's Institute nurses on an agency basis until later, when they began to recruit and employ their nursing staff directly.

The creation of the National Health Service rationalised the separate community nursing services under the local authorities, and the Medical Officers of Health were in charge of virtually all their health services, including nursing. Superintendent Nursing Officers were appointed for home nursing services (some already existed under the Queen's Institute pattern); midwives were usually managed by a head of services designated Non-Medical Supervisor of Midwives and health visitors by a Superintendent Health Visitor. However, with the growth of local authority health services provision this pattern altered, and by 1968, forty-two county councils, thirty-four county boroughs and seventeen London borough councils had appointed a Chief Nursing Officer to organise and direct the work of their community nursing services. A notable development has been the closer association of community nurses with general practitioners, resulting in improved clinical and preventive services for patients on GPs' lists. However, the single greatest hope for transforming the NHS into an integrated system of preventive care is represented in the concepts of the primary health care team and health centre practice. GPs and community nurses working in conjunction with dentists, chiropodists, social workers and others can aim to provide a comprehensive range of services to the local population, depending on the hospitals for those acute and specialist services which cannot easily be provided from a health centre. Although the development of health centres has been relatively slow, the management and organisation of community nursing services could respond to these concepts.

The Mayston Report

In 1968 the National Board for Prices and Incomes reported on the pay of nurses and midwives,[8] and it recommended implementation of the Salmon structures and salaries in the hospitals on a national scale. It also noted that the fragmented community nursing services should be coordinated by a designated head nursing officer, and this was one of the forces that motivated the DHSS to set up a working party (under the chairmanship of E.L. Mayston) to consider the extent to which the Salmon report's proposals were applicable to the community nursing services. Its report[9] was published in 1969 and commended to the local authorities by the Secretary of State. It noted that health visitors were concerned with the health of the household as a whole, health education, the early detection of abnormalities in children, the school health service and general assistance to families in difficulties. It recognised that home nurses provided skilled care under the clinical direction of GPs in patients' homes and in health centres, and recommended that they work in attachment to general practices, concentrating on rehabilitation, elementary home physiotherapy and care of the elderly and chronic sick. It also proposed that (1) every local authority should appoint a Chief Nursing Officer; (2) their senior nursing staff structure should be reviewed immediately; (3) three levels of managers (top, middle and first-line) should be appointed, and (4) management training should be provided for senior community nurses.

The result was that local authorities gradually reorganised their nursing arrangements. The title Director of Nursing Services was given to the head, and second-level 'top managers' were appointed to the larger authorities with the title Divisional Nursing Officer. Area Nursing Officers coordinated groups of nursing officers to comprise the 'middle-management' tier, leaving the qualified field workers as 'first-line managers', parallel to the Charge Nurse/Ward Sister grade of the Salmon scheme.

The Effect of the 1974 Reorganisation

The effect that the 1974 reorganisation had on the changes being instituted as a result of the Salmon and Mayston reports was one of consolidation, mainly within the districts. Its aim was, in this respect, to integrate the hospital and community nursing services and to improve the contact and cooperation between nursing and other disciplines at all levels throughout the structure. The posts of Chief Nursing Officer (Salmon) and Director of Nursing Services (Mayston) were both superseded by the creation of the District Nursing Officer (DNO) who became head of both the hospital and community nursing services. As a result, the 'top management' tasks were now handled by the District Nursing Officer and a number of Divisional Nursing Officers. These changes introduced a common hierarchy into both hospital and community nursing staff organisation for the first time. The guidance from the DHSS suggested three alternative models of organisation, and left the precise arrangements for Area Health Authorities to decide as best suited their particular circumstances.

The models were (1) a community nursing division and one or more hospital divisions, there being separate heads of each side individually responsible to the DNO; (2) functional nursing divisions reflecting 'health care groups' each managed by a division nursing officer accountable to the DNO; (3) functional nursing divisions integrating the hospital and community elements for management purposes (see Figure 27). In each case the nursing education division can serve more than one District (in multi-district areas), and district nurse and health visitor training is in any case organised on an Area basis.

The nursing staff at first-line management level and below experienced few changes as a result of the reorganisation except, perhaps, in connection with the midwifery services. At area level, the Area Nursing Officer was a member of the Area Team of Officers, and advised the Area Health Authority on all nursing matters within the Area, but did not have line-management powers over nursing services within the Districts. She was head of the nursing services provided from AHA headquarters and was closely involved in the planning process and in the establishment of close liaison with the local authority. To that extent he or she had up to five Area Nurses (depending on the Area's size and organisation) and, of course, in single-district areas, the ANO also performed the executive functions of the District Nursing Officer. The Area Nurses covered work in relation to minor capital

Figure 27 *District Nursing Organisation – Alternatives*

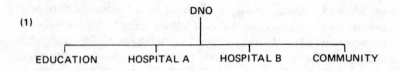

(1)

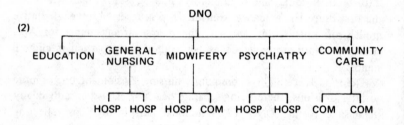

(2)

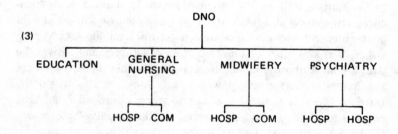

(3)

Source: Management Arrangements for the Reorganised National Health Service, HMSO, 1972

projects, services planning, personnel, local authority liaison and child health services. These posts were all administrative and advisory in content, and although their holders were highly trained and experienced nurses, they were well removed from direct contact with the care of patients. Similarly at the regional level, the Regional Nursing Officer may have some supporting Regional Nurses, and all are involved in detailed administrative work in relation to the planning and development of nursing services, professional education and personnel matters, as a vital part of the whole responsibility vested in the RHA and its staff.

One year after the reorganisation, most of the new posts that had been created for nurses were filled, and schemes of management had been drawn up. In September 1974 the report of a special committee of inquiry was published[10] recommending new rates of pay for nurses and midwives. Considerable unrest in the nursing profession, particularly on the hospital side, erupted earlier that year, over the conditions of NHS nursing work and, following unprecedented demonstrations by nursing staff, the Secretary of State set up this committee of inquiry, chaired by Lord Halsbury (who had been chairman of the Doctors' and Dentists' Review Body). The result was a substantial increase in salary for most grades of nursing staff and some increase in the holiday allowance. The Halsbury award (as it became known) was implemented by the government in late 1974 and early 1975.

Looking back, the 1970s can be seen to have faced nurses with several challenges. The 1974 reorganisation embodying the principles of Salmon and Mayston was criticised for having created an unnecessary bureaucracy. Such views were undoubtedly prejudiced and paid little regard to the managerial task of providing a continuous nursing service 24 hours a day 7 days a week. However, criticism from within nursing was not entirely absent and a preoccupation with the standard of bedside nursing led to a major reappraisal as to how this should best be organised. The nursing process, as it came to be called, concentrated less on individual disparate tasks such as dressings, feeding, giving out bedpans, and more on taking responsibility for a patient's total needs not forgetting psychological support. An RCN report *The Extended Clinical Role of the Nurse* (1979)[11] supported these moves and suggested that there should be greater professional autonomy. Following the 1974 reorganisation, Areas set up professional nursing and midwifery advisory committees whose function was to provide advice to the AHAs themselves supplementing that already received from the Area's own nursing officers, the ANO and other Area nurses and the

DNO. After 1982 the DHSS advised that such committees could continue if Districts felt them to be useful, but they were not mandatory.

As far as the organisation of nurses within Districts was concerned, the 1982 reorganisation maintained the principles of the 1974 reorganisation except that Divisions were now called Units and the Divisional Nursing Officers' titles were changed to that of Directors of Nursing Services. In recognition of the concern for improving standards of bedside nursing, the middle managers were re-designated Clinical Nurse Managers. Some District Nursing Officers have preferred the title Chief Nursing Officer. There were several other major developments during this period. The working week was reduced from 40 to 37½ hours a week; the nursing profession had to honour the EEC directives;[12] and finally and most influential, changes in training, registration and the supervision of professional standards were incorporated in the *Nurses, Midwives and Health Visitors Act* (the 1979 Act). Nurses were also having to adapt to the rapid advance of high technology medicine. Some renegotiation of responsibility, particularly between doctors and nurses, was necessary.

Education and Training

As has been said the GNC was set up in 1919 and with various amendments to its constitution remained until 1 July 1983, when it was superseded by the United Kingdom Central Council for Nursing, Midwifery and Health Visiting (UKCC), which was established by the 1979 Nurses Act. The origins of this change were largely found in the report of the *Committee on Nursing* (Briggs report)[13] which was published in 1972. The terms of reference of this committee were 'to review the role of the nurse and midwife in hospital and the community and the education and training required for that role, so that the best use is made of available manpower to meet the present needs of an integrated health service'. The recommendations were concerned with the statutory framework of nursing, with education, with manpower and conditions of work and with organisation and career structure.

The report was broadly welcomed by the profession, but it was not until May 1974 that the government responded in detail. The Secretary of State, Mrs Barbara Castle, stated in the House of Commons that the main recommendations were accepted, particularly a new pattern of education and training and a new structure of statutory bodies for the nursing and midwifery professions. She said that the age of entry would be reduced when safeguards against using students merely as 'pairs of hands' could be met. The government was aware of the health visitors' concern about a loss of identity, and agreed that the name of health visitors should be retained in the new statutory body, i.e. Central Council of Nurses, Midwives and Health Visitors, which should have a Standing Health Visiting Committee. Mrs Castle also announced that she wished to give further consideration to the structure of nursing education below national level, and to the relationship between this and the new NHS structure. She promised a future announcement about the timetable for building up adequate teaching staff and said that, in preparation, there needed to be an increase in the number of nurse tutors and clinical teachers, and a strengthening of the career structure at the level of ward sister, nurse tutor, staff nurse and equivalents. She had invited the Nurses and Midwives Whitley Council to negotiate the details within an additional expenditure of up to £18 million (3 per cent of the 1974 nurses' bill). She added that there would be consultation with the profession on what other preparatory measures could be provided within the existing statutory framework.

Accordingly, a discussion document was issued in September 1974 and various bodies within the nursing profession were asked to make their comments to the DHSS. Then in 1976 an outline of the proposals for introducing legislation to cover the sections of the Briggs report concerning the statutory framework and education was issued. In 1977 the Briggs Coordinating Committee was set up to advise on the implementation of the report's main recommendations, and in 1978 a Nurses, Midwives and Health Visitors Bill was introduced in Parliament.

This reached the statute book in 1979 and repealed the Nurses' Acts of 1957, 1964 and 1969 as well as amending a large number of clauses in other Acts concerned with nurses, midwives and health visitors. The 1979 Act set up the UKCC which from 1 July 1983, became responsible for the following tasks: establishing and improving standards of training and professional conduct, determining rules for registration and maintaining a single professional register, giving guidance to the profession on standards of professional conduct, and protecting the public from unsafe practitioners.

The UKCC has 45 members of whom 17 are appointed direct by the Secretary of State and the remaining 28 are nominated by the National Boards, 7 from each. The National Boards for England, Wales, Scotland and Northern Ireland are statutory bodies in their own right and responsible for implementing policies and rules decided by the UKCC. In particular they have to provide, or arrange for others to provide, courses of training leading to regulation and further postgraduate training at approved institutions. They have to ensure that courses meet the requirements of the UKCC, and must hold, or arrange to be held, examinations in connection with these courses. They also collaborate with the UKCC on promoting improved training and carry out investigations of alleged misconduct prior to referral to the UKCC Professional Conduct Committee (who have powers to remove a nurse, midwife or health visitor from the register).

The UKCC has a number of statutory standing committees concerned with finance, educational policy, research, registration and professional conduct. Three of the committees recognise the special interests of midwifery, district nursing and health visiting. (Failure to give due recognition to the different traditions of these three aspects of nursing delayed the discussion of the bill through Parliament.) The National Boards also have statutory sub-committees for finance and midwifery and in practice have also set up other sub-committees, for instance, for mental illness and mental handicap nursing. The English National Board felt this to be in the spirit of observing the 1979 Act's requirement to 'have proper regard for the interest of all groups within the profession, including those with minority representation'.

An important change following the 1979 Act was the new rules for training and registration. The minimum age for entry to nursing has been lowered to 17½, although National Boards may maintain the 18 year rule if they wish. From 1 January 1986 there will be a minimum educational requirement for all first level entrants of five 'O' level passes or success in the UKCC special test. The term 'first level' needs explanation. We have seen that assistant nurses were first accepted for training following the 1943 Nurses Act. The Briggs report discussed the concept of a 'common portal of entry' whereby those intending to nurse would have a common period of study specialising only after the core course. This proposal worried many who felt that the entry requirements would either be too low for clinical nurses with high academic qualifications or too high for those who were wishing to become good practical nurses. The new rules present a compromise by having one professional register recognising within it first and second level entrants. The new register merges all the previous registers, rolls and records maintained by nine separate bodies into a single register with eleven parts. The aim is to provide a single computerised record of all nurses giving a data set of personal details, training courses undertaken and resulting qualifications.

It is too early to assess how radical the 1979 Act was. For instance, it is not yet clear whether the Briggs report concept of student status for nurses in training will be developed to the point where it replaces the traditional 'apprentice' role of the trainee. This would result in wards being covered by trained and untrained staff with nurses in training as a supernumerary element. Whatever the future, the 1979 Act stands as a major piece of legislation bringing together the various elements of nursing for the first time under one professional body.

One other event should not be passed without comment. The Committee of Enquiry into Mental Handicap Nursing and Care 1979 (Jay report, referred to in Chapter 7 in the discussion on mental handicap) challenged the basic assumption that traditional nurse training, even with its special syllabus for the mentally handicapped, was appropriate for those working in this field. The report suggested that the Certificate in Social Service was a more appropriate qualification. A determined campaign against these proposals, their likely cost, the setting up of the UKCC which was already going through Parliament, and the 1982 reorganisation all worked against any significant progress being made in this matter. However, the gradual resettlement of mentally handicapped people in the community still leaves the question of appropriate training for those concerned with them an open issue.

Nurses in Management

Nurses in the United Kingdom have higher managerial status than elsewhere in the world where they are subordinate to either doctor managers or general managers. The position could change and to end this chapter the role of nurses in management is reviewed. The matron of a voluntary hospital and, after 1929, of the municipal hospital, had a unique status. Not only did she (men were not involved until after the Second World War) look after all nursing staff, but she was also concerned with other housekeeping duties including the cleaning, catering and linen services. To help her there were assistant matrons, housekeeping and home sisters who were not generally perceived as part of the nursing hierarchy. The tradition of one manager and one decision maker, much quoted in later years, was thus created. Following the introduction of the NHS the matron's role began to change. Progressively through the 1950s general administrators took over the non-nursing duties. The tradition of unmarried women as matrons (former Poor Law hospitals however had matrons who were married) gradually disappeared. Shorter hours for nurses allowed hospitals to change from having just one matron living in and always on call. By the 1960s it was felt that the role of nurses in the management structure should be examined. The Salmon report did much for nurses as managers, but it also had its detractors. Doctors and administrators found the apparent increase in nursing bureaucracy frustrating. Direct contacts with either the ward sister or the matron were now obscured by the proliferation of ranks of Nursing Officers, Senior Nursing Officers and Principal Nursing Officers. Nurses themselves were not entirely in support of the new system, particularly those who wished to remain in the clinical field. They found that nurses promoted into management jobs overtook them in status and salary. A ward sister's loyalty is always somewhat divided between the nursing hierarchy on the one hand and the consultant medical staff with whom she works on the other. The new structure aggravated this situation.

The 1974 reorganisation increased nurses' involvement in management, particularly at Area level where there were few opportunities for clinical nursing. Planning and personnel matters absorbed the Area Nursing Officer and his or her staff. This duplicated effort within Districts to a certain extent and tension between the two developed. Within Districts the development of sector management gave some degree of corporate responsibility to Divisional Nursing Officers (previously Principal Nursing Officers). At DMT level this involvement in the running of the District as a whole was a significant development in the managerial responsibility for the District Nursing Officer.

The 1982 reorganisation seemed to confirm nurses' management role with the formation of units presided over by an administrator, a nurse and a doctor acting as a triumvirate. The Griffiths report questioned this arrangement and the Royal College of Nursing was most vehement in its criticisms of the proposals, not only because it felt that the right of nurses to manage nurses was under attack, but also because it believed the concept of the general manager was likely to reduce the managerial status of those nurses on Unit and District management teams. It seemed unlikely that faced with the claims of administrators and doctors for this role that nurses themselves would often become general managers. Whatever the outcome of these proposals for reform, a nursing presence in the top levels of management would seem to be desirable. At this level there is the dual responsibility of managing a large set of resources and maintaining the 24 hour care of patients of all kinds within an increasingly rigorous set of professional standards.

Notes

1. Quoted in: A.M. Carr-Saunders and P.A. Wilson, *The Professions*, Cass, London, 1933, p. 118 (from Elizabeth Haldane, *The British Nurse in Peace and War*, 1923).

2. *Local Government Act, 1929*, 19 Geo. 5, Ch. 17, HMSO, London, 1929.

3. Ministry of Health and Scottish Home and Health Department. *Report of the Committee on Senior Nursing Staff Structure* (Chairman, B. Salmon), HMSO, London, 1966.

4. *Report of a Working Party in the Field of Work, Training and Recruitment of Health Visitors* (Jamieson Report), HMSO, London, 1956.

5. Quoted in: A.M. Carr-Saunders and P.A. Wilson op. cit., p. 122 (from Emma Brierly, *In the Beginning*, 1924).

6. Ministry of Health. *Report of the Maternity Services Committee* (Cranbrook Report), HMSO, London, 1959.

7. Central Health Services Council. *Domiciliary Midwifery and Maternity Bed Needs* (Peel Report), HMSO, London, 1970.

8. National Board for Prices and Incomes. *Pay of Nurses and Midwives in the National Health Service*, Report No. 60, HMSO, London, 1968 (Cmnd. 3585).

9. Department of Health and Social Security. Scottish Home and Health Department. Welsh Office. *Report of the Working Party on Management Structures in the Local Authority Nursing Services* (Chairman, E.L. Mayston), 1969.

10. Department of Health and Social Security. *Report of the Committee of Inquiry into Pay and Related Conditions of Service of Nurses and Midwives* (Chairman, Lord Halsbury), HMSO, London, 1974 (Supplement to the Report published in 1975).

11. Royal College of Nursing of the United Kingdom. *The Extended Clinical Role of the Nurse*, RCN, London, 1979.

12. Britain's membership of the European Community made certain reforms necessary: the 1977 Directives specified that length of training should in future be counted in hours rather than years and that all nursing recruits should have at least 10 years general education. No attempt was made to introduce a nursing qualification that was common throughout the Community.

13. *Report of the Committee on Nursing* (Chairman, Professor Asa Briggs), HMSO, London, 1972 (Cmnd. 5115).

10 OTHER STAFF

In addition to doctors and nurses, the NHS employs many other groups of staff (see Figure 28 for the distribution of broad categories). Some of these are independent practitioners but most are directly employed. Both types will be described in this chapter.

Figure 28 *NHS Staff* (whole-time equivalents, England, in thousands)

	1978	1979	1980	1981	1982	1983 (Provisional)
Medical and dental[2] (hospital and community)	36	37	38	39	39	40
Nursing and Midwifery[3]	351	358	370[4]	392	397	397
Professional and technical	57	60	62	65	67	39
Works	6	6	6	6	6	6
Maintenance	20	20	21	21	21	21
Administrative and clerical	100	103	105	109	109	110
Ambulance (incl. officers)	17	17	18	18	18	18
Ancillary	172	172	172	172	171	166
Total	760[1]	773	792	822	829	827

1. Figures rounded and therefore may not sum to the totals.
2. Excludes hospital practitioners, part-time medical officers (clinical assistants) general medical practitioners participating in Hospital Staff Funds and occasional sessional staff in the community health services. Includes locums.
3. Includes agency nurses and midwives and health visitor students. Excludes student nurses (community).
4. In 1980 the working week for nursing and midwifery staff was reduced from 40 to 37½ hours. Approximately half the increase in staff in that year is estimated to be attributable to the need to employ more to counteract the reduction in total man-hours available.
Source: The Government's Expenditure Plans 1983/4–1986/7 (Cmnd. 9143) 1984

Dental Services

In the seventeenth and eighteenth centuries there was no distinct profession of dentistry, but some barber-surgeons became known as 'operators for the teeth'. As scientific study of the teeth advanced, some practitioners were able to become very skilled specialists while others, who remained unskilled and unqualified, obtained their work through advertising. In 1878 the Dentists Act empowered the General Medical Council to examine and register suitable qualified dentists, but unqualified dentists continued to practice. The British Dental Association was founded in 1880 and dentistry became recognised as a profession. Unregistered practitioners continued to flourish, and many of them were inadequately trained, but it was not until 1921 that a new Dentists Act dealt with this by effectively closing the profession to anyone who was not trained at a school of dentistry recognised by the newly created Dental Board. The Act made the Dental Board responsible for keeping a register and for investigating cases of misconduct, but the GMC retained control over disciplinary action and the power to license practitioners.

A further Dentists Act in 1957 established the General Dental Council as the single statutory licensing and registering body which took on the functions of the Dental Board and the GMC (in relation to dentistry). It supervises the standard of dental examinations and teaching and keeps the register of dentists who have obtained the professional qualifications — either a degree (Bachelor of Dental Surgery, BDS) or a diploma (Licentiate in Dental Surgery, LDS) — from an approved school of dentistry. The training takes between four and six years, and dentists pay an entry and retention fee to have their name on the register. Practitioners' names can be erased if they commit a felony or if they are found guilty of professional misconduct by the Council's disciplinary committee. The Dentists Act 1983 revised the membership of the Council. There are now twenty-nine members, of whom eighteen are registered dentists elected from amongst themselves, four are the chief dental officers from England, Wales, Scotland and Northern Ireland, six are lay people nominated by the Queen on the advice of the Privy Council and one is a dental auxiliary. The President is elected from this membership. In addition three members of the General Medical Council can join discussions on dental education and examination issues. Those universities with dental schools can also send one member each (two for the University of London) who are additional to the twenty-nine members and must themselves be dentists.

Dental Services before 1974

Before the NHS was founded, the general state of dental health was very poor, and although dental benefits were available under the National Health Insurance scheme to thirteen million of the working

population, only about six per cent made claims. After 1948, the NHS
provided dental services in each arm of the tripartite structure. Hospital
dentists specialised in dental surgery or orthodontics (the straightening
of children's teeth) and were graded in the same way as hospital
medical staff. Some worked in dental departments of general hospitals
and others worked within specialist dental hospitals. Local authorities
were obliged by the 1944 Education Act to provide free dental inspection and treatment for all children in maintained schools, and they also
cared for the dental health of expectant and nursing mothers. In fact
the School Medical Service, established in 1907, made provision for
dental care of the mothers and children of pre-school age, but less than
two per cent of the eligible population made use of this. The explicit
aim of the local authority dental services was to conserve teeth and
to prevent premature loss of first teeth in children. The services were
organised by a Principal School Dental Officer (responsible to the
Medical Officer of Health) and his staff of School Dental Officers
worked in the schools, clinics and treatment centres run by the local
authority.

Then as now the largest sector of the dental services was provided by
dentists in general practice. These were qualified registered dentists
who worked from their own homes or other premises, obtained their
own equipment and supplies, and employed ancillary staff. They held
contracts with the Executive Councils which paid them for treating
patients under the NHS. Many combined this with private practice,
and they were not obliged to undertake any more NHS work than they
wished.

Dental Services since 1974

In 1974, the reorganisation only changed the administration of dental
services; it did not alter this pattern of clinical work. Hospital dental
surgeons (consultant oral surgeons and orthodontists) remained employees of the RHAs (or, in the case of Teaching Areas, the AHA(T)),
and junior dental staff were employed by the Districts. Local authority
dental staff were transferred to the new Areas which became
responsible for community and school dental services throughout
the Area. General dental practitioners remained in contract with the
FPCs. The 1982 reorganisation fragmented these arrangements by
devolving the Area responsibilities to each District which appointed
a District Dental Officer accountable to the DHA. Dental Advisory
Committees ceased to be statutory in 1982 but most Districts have
set one up. These committees exist to give expert opinion on the

provision of dental services; they are not concerned with the relations between the profession and its employers or with the internal organisation of the profession.

Dentists' Pay

As with doctors, dentists have one body to represent them professionally (the British Dental Association), one statutory body to regulate and control their practice (the General Dental Council) and separate bodies to negotiate their pay. Since 1960 their pay has been determined by the permanent review body which was established following the recommendations of the Royal Commission on Doctors' and Dentists' Remuneration.[1] Since 1974, community dentists have also become NHS employees and their pay has therefore also come within the scope of the review body. Hospital and community dental staff receive a salary from their health authority but the system for general dental practitioners is more complicated.

Before 1948, general dental practitioners received most of their income from private practice, and a committee[2] was appointed to work out a scheme for paying them under the NHS. It fixed a target net income for the average weekly chairside hours being worked, and the Health Departments and the profession jointly worked out fees for different items of service that should provide this level of income. However, the initial demand for dentures and dental treatment was enormous, so dentists worked more hours and received higher incomes than had been anticipated. The government imposed limits on top earnings and charges for dentures were introduced in 1951. Demand gradually declined, but because full information about dentists' total earnings (i.e. including private practice) and practice expenses was not available, the Health Departments and the BDA jointly discussed how to fix future levels of remuneration. The BDA demanded removal of the limit on top earnings, but the Department was insistent, although it suggested new rates for items of service which could raise the ceiling for top incomes. The BDA was not enthusiastic about this, but a survey of its members showed that a majority were not against this system of payment, so it accepted. The Royal Commission on Doctors' and Dentists' Remuneration made some specific recommendations about the pay of dentists, and it confirmed that general dental practitioners' pay should be based on fees for items of service.

The Doctors' and Dentists' Review Body advised the government on the average net income that dentists should receive for working a specified number of chairside hours per year. The Dental Rates Study

Group (a committee of representatives from the profession and the DHSS under an independent Chairman) assesses from time to time the level of dentists' practice expenses from information provided by the Inland Revenue in order to determine average gross earnings, and hence to draw up a scale of fees to produce average earnings of that level. The effect of this system is gradually to reduce the fee for a given treatment as more of those treatments are being carried out faster or more efficiently. The system has been called 'the treadmill' because it rewards dentists for doing a greater number of those treatments. It tends to reward restorative work (fillings) rather than preventive treatment. The costs of general dental services to the NHS are therefore controlled to some extent by the degree of accuracy of the Dental Rates Study Group's calculations. The Dental Estimates Board has to give prior approval for discretionary fees which can be claimed for treatments where a range of possible costs exists. Its records indicate the number and range of different courses of treatment that are given under the NHS, but no comparable figures exist for the extent of private treatment and for the number of people who do not go to a dentist at all.

These arrangements create a direct link between the number of patients seen and the pay of dentists. It is not altogether surprising therefore that in 1983 the BDA issued a document[3] attacking the rise in dental charges. Using data from the Office of Population Censuses and Surveys, the BDA pointed out that those patients who only attended a dentist in an emergency had 3.3 more missing teeth and 1.9 more decayed teeth, than regular attenders. The BDA claimed that the disproportionate rise in dental charges would deter patients from regular visits to their dentists. Broadly speaking the charges had risen by more than double the rate of inflation. In the five years ending in 1983, the patients' share of dental costs had increased from 17 per cent to 27 per cent with a corresponding reduction in direct exchequer funding. Such problems do not usually affect the hospital or community dental services where charges are not made for treatment. Charges are payable for dentures and other appliances which would otherwise be obtained from a general dental practitioner.

Dental Manpower

Regional variations in the distribution of dentists have always been marked, and are associated with the social class structure, such that there tend to be proportionally more dentists in areas with proportionally more people in the higher social classes. In order to strengthen the professional manpower, some observers favour greater use of dental auxiliaries. These staff work with general dental practitioners, dealing with all the administrative duties as well as preparing instruments, mixing fillings materials and processing X-rays. Dental hygienists are trained in schools of dentistry to be able to clean, scale and polish teeth, and they also play an important part in giving advice to patients about dental hygiene. In the school dental service, dental therapists are people trained to carry out simple fillings, extract milk teeth, and clean, scale and polish the teeth of school children, and also teach them about the importance of proper oral hygiene. Although the number of auxiliary staff is small (their remuneration is negotiated through Professional and Technical Whitley Council 'B') they can clearly take on the routine work under supervision and allow the dentist to apply his specialist skills and knowledge more widely. The General Dental Council controls their professional conduct through a sub-committee, the Dental Auxiliaries Committee. Dental technicians are needed to make dentures, crowns, inlays and other appliances. They serve an apprenticeship in a dental laboratory, a hospital or a commercial firm, or can undergo full-time training. Many general dental practitioners use the services of a commercial laboratory but in hospital departments technicians also do work in connection with the treatment of facial injuries.

Ophthalmic Services

The Worshipful Company of Spectacle Makers was given a Royal Charter in 1629, and opticians date their professional origins back to this time. However, it was not until the mid-nineteenth century that instruments for examining the eye and investigating refractive errors were invented, thus enabling the scientific diagnosis and treatment of sight disorders to develop. Qualified doctors specialising in the study of the eye took on the work of sight testing as did the opticians who also sold spectacles. In 1895 the British Optical Association was founded, its aim being to achieve state registration for opticians, which would eliminate unqualified practitioners and establish professional status for the duly qualified. In 1923, a register of the Joint Council of Qualified Opticians was instituted, and the Council promoted a bill for state registration. But the BMA were against it since they regarded doctors as being exclusively qualified to detect disease, and stated that all sight testing should be carried out under medical supervision. Most of the approved societies under the National Health Insurance scheme required the people they covered to go only to a practitioner on this register or to a doctor for sight testing.

At the time of the introduction of the NHS there were several different groups testing sight and supplying spectacles, and they possessed varying standards of professional qualification. In order to regularise the situation it was decided to place all sight testing in the hospital sector under specialist doctors (called ophthalmologists) while the dispensing of spectacles could go on inside or outside the hospitals. However, since the hospitals in 1948 were not able to take on the full service a Supplementary Ophthalmic Service was instituted.[4] It allowed for ophthalmic medical practitioners and ophthalmic opticians to continue as independent operators, placing them under contracts with the NHS administered through the Executive Councils. But the intended shift to a hospital service never happened and in the Health Service and Public Health Act 1968,[5] the word 'supplementary' was removed, and the name changed to General Ophthalmic Service. Ophthalmic medical practitioners only test sight and prescribe lenses, ophthalmic opticians test sight and prescribe and dispense lenses to their patients, and dispensing opticians supply spectacles and contact lenses prescribed by ophthalmic medical practitioners or ophthalmic opticians. Most of the work is done in the community, although orthoptists, who treat squints in children, work entirely in hospitals. Under the school health service, sight testing is provided for children, but if treatment is required they have to attend a hospital or consult an optician.

In 1953 the Crook report[6] recommended a General Optical Council should be established to maintain a register of ophthalmic and dispensing opticians, and to exercise governing and disciplinary powers over them. This was accepted by the government but it was not until 1958 that the Council was established under the Opticians Act, partly because of strong opposition by sections of the medical profession. The General Optical Council gave opticians their independent professional status and restricted the legal prescribing of dispensing of spectacles to them (or registered medical practitioners). The necessary qualifications for registration of ophthalmic opticians are granted after three years full-time study by the Worshipful Company, the British Optical Association and the Institute of Ophthalmic Science. Dispensing opticians can obtain qualifications for registration through two years full-time study, three years day release or four years correspondence course, from the Association of Dispensing Opticians or with the Dispensing Certificate of the British Optical Association. Most dispensing opticians are members of the National Ophthalmic Treatment Board (NOTB) Association, and practise from medical eye centres that this body monitors.

As with dental services, the demand for ophthalmic services at the start of the NHS was very high, and it appeared that removing the barrier of cost enabled many people who needed spectacles to come forward and obtain them. Opticians' pay is negotiated through the Optical Whitley Council although most of them dispense non-NHS lenses and frames as well. An optician does not have a list of patients like a GP, but is paid a separate fee for each item of service, under the terms of his contract with the Family Practitioner Committee. Patients also pay a charge for lenses and frames, and these payments virtually cover the cost of them to the optician. Ophthalmic and dispensing opticians obtain spectacles made up to their specification from prescription houses, at prices fixed by negotiations between the DHSS and the prescription houses and set out in the 'Statement of Fees and Charges'.[7] Prescription houses purchase lenses and frames from manufacturing firms either unfinished or in semi-finished form, and fit the lenses to the frames according to prescriptions placed with them by the opticians. Some of the dispensing opticians' businesses are owned by multiple chains, some of which also own prescription houses. Non-NHS frames are very popular, and NHS lenses can be fitted to them although they cost the patient and the optician more to obtain. Similarly, if an optician dispenses private lenses and frames, his fee will be higher than under the NHS, and it will be borne by the patient.

These arrangements were challenged at the end of 1983 by a new Bill in Parliament which embodied the government's intention to remove the monopoly from opticians and allow spectacles to be supplied by any retailer. This move was stimulated by the belief that the monopoly had kept the cost of non-NHS frames and lenses unduly high, particularly when compared to other countries. However the proposal went much further and abolished the supply of NHS frames and lenses to all but children and certain people on low incomes. Although consumer representatives initially welcomed these reforms because of the opportunity to buy spectacles at a lower price, the ophthalmic profession was highly critical. They said it would mean many people needing spectacles would obtain them without an eye test thus endangering their sight and even their own and other people's safety. This change in policy was one outcome of the government review of ophthalmic services set up earlier in 1983. The terms of reference also included a review of the structure of the service and methods of remuneration. Until that time the ophthalmic service had been very stable for a variety of reasons. First, apart from the development of plastic, multifocal and contact lenses, there have been no major technical advances in the production of spectacle lenses. Secondly, over the age of forty-five, an increasingly large section of the population needs to wear spectacles. Thirdly, the manufacturing process for NHS lenses is basically unchanged, so that increased production costs have been less than increases in manufacturing costs in general. This stability has helped the NHS considerably because the constant and wide demand for spectacles can be met by opticians who can extend their incomes through non-NHS work. The NHS has therefore been able to provide an adequate comprehensive service that is not fully integrated with the medical services, yet the existence of demand for private treatment has made it worthwhile for opticians to undertake NHS work as well.

Opticians have a representative body called the Local Optical Committee. The post-1974 Statutory Area Advisory Committee was superseded in 1982 by an optional District Optical Committee with a membership of ophthalmic and dispensing opticians representative of both the general Ophthalmic Services and the Hospital Eye Service. DHSS advice also allowed for a Regional Optical Committee.[8]

Pharmaceutical Services

The pharmacists' profession can also trace its origins back three or four hundred years, but it developed from two distinct lines. The Society of Apothecaries was founded in 1617, and its members dispensed medicines on the order of physicians as well as prescribing and dispensing medicines for patients themselves; the chemists and druggists were retail shopkeepers who did not prescribe, but prepared and sold medicines in competition with the apothecaries. The Apothecaries Act of 1815 allowed apothecaries to charge for their professional advice to patients as well as for the medicines they dispensed, and this encouraged them to become more like general medical practitioners. The chemists and druggists progressively took over as the dispensers of physicians' prescriptions. The Pharmaceutical Society of Great Britain was formed in 1841, and the Pharmacy Acts of 1852 and 1868 gave it the statutory duty to register pharmaceutical chemists who had obtained its diploma after training and examination, and to prevent those who were not pharmaceutical chemists or chemists or druggists from dispensing medicines or selling poisons. Under the National Health Insurance scheme only registered pharmacists could dispense medicines prescribed for insured people (except in remote areas where the doctors themselves could dispense their prescriptions).

Under the National Health Service, separate arrangements are made for dispensing medicines in the hospitals and the community. The Hospital Pharmaceutical Service employs registered pharmacists and technicians to prepare and dispense medicines to hospital inpatients and outpatients as prescribed by hospital doctors. The General Pharmaceutical Service involves retail pharmacists in dispensing medicines prescribed by general practitioners, under contract with the Family Practitioner Committees (Executive Councils before 1974). In 1974 AHAs appointed Area Pharmaceutical Officers to supervise the hospital pharmaceutical services even though each District probably had a District Pharmacist. After 1982 DHSS advice left DHAs to decide on the status and role of the head of the hospital pharmaceutical services, but most, if not all, Districts have appointed a District Pharmaceutical Officer who reports either to the District Administrator or the District Medical Officer but has direct access to the DMT and the DHA. Most Districts have a District Pharmaceutical Committee to advise on developments and on matters such as compliance with the Medicines Act and the formulation of drug use guidelines to ensure that money is not wasted on proprietory brands where a cheaper generic substitute would be as effective. Most Regions also have some sort of Regional advisory machinery.

The General Pharmaceutical Service

The system of providing general pharmaceutical services under the NHS exists to provide patients free of charge (subject to a nominal prescription charge for some categories of patients) with drugs and appliances that have been prescribed by their doctors for them. The system is also designed to impose a number of controls which will contain the costs of drugs within reasonable limits. Doctors are free to prescribe any drugs and appliances (but not foods or toiletries) which will, in their opinion, benefit the health of their patients. They write out the prescription on a standard form which is taken to a chemist for dispensing, or sometimes is dispensed by the doctor. The chemist supplies the prescribed drugs from stocks which he has purchased from the manufacturers or a wholesaler. He pays the supplier on normal credit terms, and is reimbursed by the Family Practitioner Committee for the prescriptions he has dispensed. At the end of each month the chemist sends the prescription forms to the Prescription Pricing Authority which calculates the costs of the ingredients according to the Drug Tariff. This is a list of the prices of drugs which is issued annually by the DHSS together with amendments during the year. For each prescription, the Prescription Pricing Authority also calculates the on-cost allowance for the chemist's overhead expenses and profits, his dispensing fee and an allowance for containers. It then notifies the Family Practitioner Committee of the amount to be paid to the chemist for the month's prescriptions.

The Prescription Pricing Authority came into existence in 1974 to continue the work that had been carried out since 1948 by the Joint Pricing Committee, and before that by Joint Pricing Bureaux under the National Health Insurance Scheme. Its main offices are in Newcastle-upon-Tyne and there are eight other offices in the north of England which each price the NHS prescriptions for specified parts of England. The Authority has eight members nominated from the FPCs, and the DHSS nominates one doctor and three pharmacists. It has almost 2,000 staff who process about 275 million prescriptions annually. In Wales the Welsh Health Technical Services Organisation does this pricing work for the FPCs.

The Prescription Pricing Authority also uses the information from a sample of prescriptions it prices in order to prepare estimates of drug use by therapeutic group, class of preparation, etc. and to give indications of the number of prescriptions submitted and the average cost per prescription each month. In addition, once every year each general practitioner is sent a statement of the number and cost of the prescriptions he has issued during one month. From these calculations the average costs of all doctors in that FPC area can be compared with that individual doctor's costs.

In 1976 an inquiry into the work of the Prescription Pricing Authority was initiated because of concern over delays in paying the accounts of chemist contractors and dispensing doctors, and because of difficulties in obtaining information about prescribing patterns in order to tackle the problem of the cost of the pharmaceutical services. The report of the inquiry was published in January 1977[9] making a number of short-term recommendations for speeding up the settlement of accounts. It also suggested that the Authority should give doctors information about their prescribing patterns, and give more information generally to the DHSS, the Committee on Safety of Medicines and the pharmaceutical industry.

If a chemist (who may be an individual, a firm or a corporate body) wishes to open a shop as a pharmacy, he first has to have the premises registered in accordance with the Medicines Act 1968, and this is done through the mediation of the Pharmaceutical Society of Great Britain. A pharmacist who wishes to dispense NHS medicines then has to apply to the FPC for a contract which specifies the terms and conditions of service, and includes requirements relating to opening hours and participation in the out-of-hours rota service. If a pharmacist wishes to have different opening hours from those specified he has to apply to the Hours of Service Committee of the FPC. This committee specifies the minimum opening hours and the rota service that chemists are obliged to observe, and keeps these arrangements and any special cases under review. Pay negotiations for retail pharmacists are handled by the Pharmaceutical Whitley Council, and their central representative body is the Pharmaceutical Services Negotiating Committee. The National Pharmaceutical Union was founded in 1920 as a trade association for individual retail pharmacists. In recent years it has changed its brief to include the interests of employee pharmacists, and has also admitted company chemists to membership — this group now forms the majority of its members and it has changed its name to the National Pharmaceutical Association.

A chemist is only likely to open a shop on a given site if the balance of NHS work and over-the-counter sales he could expect there would be economically worthwhile. As a result, pharmacies have been closing at the rate of approximately 300 each year, and comprehensive pharmaceutical coverage throughout England and Wales has been jeopardised. For a number of years a 'rural area subsidy' payment had been available to certain chemists in order to preserve services to rural communities, but this was not able to prevent closures. However, in 1977 after protracted discussions between the DHSS and the Pharmaceutical Services Negotiating Committee, a new system called the 'Essential Small Pharmacies Scheme' was implemented. It provides for supplementary payments to be made to pharmacies which are 3 kilometres or more from the nearest pharmacy, dispense between 6,000 and 30,000 prescriptions annually, have a non-NHS turnover of less than £25,000 per annum (at March 1976 prices) and provide a full pharmaceutical service. It has also been agreed that pharmacies which do not meet these stringent criteria but are also in difficulties will in future be considered for extra payments under the new scheme.

The Relationship between the NHS and the Pharmaceutical Industry

The number of prescriptions is enormous. In 1982 approximately 311 million prescriptions were dispensed at a total cost of £1,180 million. This is an average of £3.79 per prescription and seven prescriptions per person per year. In view of the large costs, every government has shown considerable interest in controlling expenditure on drugs. The pharmaceutical companies in turn aim their sales promotion efforts at the doctors because doctors decide which medicines to prescribe. Under the arrangements which have been described, neither the doctor nor the patient pays for the medicines (the prescription charge paid by patients represents only a portion of the prescription cost — about 37 per cent in 1983). Ministers are responsible to Parliament for their departments' spending of Exchequer funds and from the earliest days of the NHS successive health ministers have been under pressure from the Public Accounts Committee to ensure that prices paid to pharmaceutical companies are reasonable. The problem is that the companies sell most of their pharmaceuticals in the UK to the National Health Services since there is comparatively little non-NHS prescribing. The pharmaceutical industry has insisted that it needs a high level of profitability in order to finance research and to cover the high risks in developing new drugs. Over the years a number of attempts to control the cost of prescribed medicines have been made by successive governments. In 1949 the Joint Committee on the Classification of Proprietary Preparations was set up by the Central and Scottish Health Services Councils to advise the health ministers on the status of proprietary preparations and to indicate where less expensive standard forms of these preparations existed.

The point was that pharmaceutical manufacturers market certain medicines under brand names to ensure continuity of sales if they are the originator of the product, or to distinguish their formulation from similar ones of the same basic chemicals. Often, therapeutically identical unbranded (or non-proprietary) preparations can be obtained at lower cost. The Joint Committee's classification (which was periodically revised) together with the British National Formulary, the British Pharmacopaeia, the British Pharmaceutical Codex, Data Sheets and Prescribers' Notes all provide listings which are intended to guide doctors away from the expensive proprietary medicines wherever a standard and less expensive alternative exists. The Hinchliffe Committee[10] was set up in 1957 to investigate the cost of prescribing and it recommended that where a GP habitually exceeded the local average for prescription costs (as shown in returns from the pricing offices to the Executive Councils) the Local Medical Committee should investigate the case. Penalties imposed on GPs for overprescribing should be severe. In fact, a negligible number of GPs have been investigated by LMCs, the highest penalty being in the region of £100. Since 1971 no penalties have been imposed, although some GPs (about 2,000 in 1974) are visited by Regional Medical Officers of the DHSS to discuss the pattern and cost of their prescribing.

Another facet of the pharmaceutical industry's relationship with the NHS is that most of the research and clinical trials on new products are controlled by the manufacturers and not the consumers. Few medicines that are introduced can be entirely free from risks and preparatory testing for safety is required before general issue. The Committee on Safety of Drugs (Chairman, Sir Derrick Dunlop) was set up in 1963 to monitor the process of testing used by the industry before its products could be allowed on the market. In 1964 the Joint Committee was dissolved while the Dunlop Committee remained to regulate the safety of drugs. A new committee was also set up (Chairman, Sir Alastair McGregor) to classify medicines into therapeutic categories, and thus to advise practitioners on whether, in the Committee's expert view, particular drugs were worth using.

As well as influencing the prescribing habits of doctors, governments have also attempted to determine fair prices for their NHS drug purchases, and in 1958 a Voluntary Price Regulation Scheme (VPRS) was negotiated with the industry, which related the price of prescribed medicines to their prices in overseas markets (on the assumption that where patients or private insurance companies had to pay for the medicines, the prices were likely to be reasonable).[11] Continued pressure from the Public Accounts Committee to reduce the NHS drugs bill and political concern over the incidence of price fixing by manufacturers of patented medicines brought about negotiations for a second VPRS in 1961. This established that the prices of major products should be the subject of direct price negotiations on the basis of the supplying companies' overall profitability. In 1964 and 1972, further modifications to the VPRS were negotiated. However, these arrangements did not cover all the products purchased by the NHS and there were significant problems in isolating those profits resulting solely from the UK pharmaceutical trading of international companies. In 1977, after further negotiations between the government and the pharmaceutical industry, a new agreement was reached: the Pharmaceutical Price Regulation Scheme (PPRS), which superseded the VPRS. Under the new arrangements, more stringent controls have been imposed on the contents of drug advertisements, the manufacturers are obliged to submit forecasts of profitability of medicines sales to the NHS before the end of the financial year (thus improving the ability of the government to check unacceptably high profits), and the government's power to obtain compulsory licensing of pharmaceutical patents has been removed.

An event that shocked the pharmaceutical industry occurred in 1961 when it became known that some hospital pharmacists had been buying cheaper but chemically identical supplies from unlicensed manufacturers in countries which did not operate schemes for granting patents to pharmaceutical products.[12] Technically the pharmacists were breaking the law (although they were saving money for the NHS), so the Minister of Health (Enoch Powell) decided to invoke Section 46 of the Patents Act 1948, which legalised these imports for 'the services of the Crown' in relation to hospital pharmaceutical supplies. In 1965, the government discontinued these imports in return for satisfactory price settlements between regular UK suppliers and the NHS. Nevertheless, the government's wish to rationalise the form of its negotiations with the manufacturing companies and its concern to control the continually rising costs of pharmaceuticals resulted in the setting up of the Committee of Inquiry into the Relationship of the Pharmaceutical Industry and the National Health Service in 1965 (the Sainsbury Committee).[13] Its report, published two years later, contained four major recommendations:

(1) Companies should provide annual financial returns to the Ministry of Health showing in prescribed form the returns from its pharmaceutical business;
(2) Problems associated with financial transfers and transactions with associated companies should be controlled;
(3) Companies should submit 'Standard Cost Returns' showing proposed prices and costs for new products, and eventually for major products already on the market;
(4) A Medicines Commission should be set up.

Points 1 and 2 were accepted and taken up in discussion between the industry and the NHS on further revisions of the VPRS. Point 3 was rejected by the Association of the British Pharmaceutical Industry (the representative body for pharmaceutical manufacturers) on the grounds that because of the high costs of innovation, operating ratios could only be reviewed as a whole rather than in relation to individual products. The Ministry of Health also made it clear that they would not have enough civil servants of suitable ability to scrutinise these returns.

The Medicines Act was passed in 1968 and embodies the Sainsbury recommendation for a Medicines Commission. This has replaced the Dunlop Committee and under it a new Committee on the Safety of Medicines has been set up. The Act completely recast the legal basis for research, manufacture and development of medicinal products.[14]

Although all these steps represent a considerable effort to regularise the supply and prescription of pharmaceuticals under the NHS, the apparently incompatible requirements of governments and the industry make it difficult for smooth negotiations on prices to be maintained. The pharmaceutical industry is more profitable than industry as a whole: in the UK, about 14 per cent return on money invested is the average for all industry while the pharmaceutical sector achieves an average return of 25 per cent. The industry maintains that this profit is earned by its efficiency and is a necessary buffer to the high risk factor, but critics reply that patented brand names and heavy sales promotions give the manufacturers quasi-monopolistic powers. The situation can be illustrated by the case of Hoffmann-La Roche.

Hoffmann-La-Roche is a Swiss-based pharmaceutical company which developed two particularly successful tranquillisers, marketed in the UK by its operating company Roche Products Ltd, under the brand names Valium and Librium. By 1970 Valium and Librium accounted for 68 per cent of all tranquillisers prescribed under the NHS and, since they were relatively highly priced, the company was able to make substantial profits on these sales. Roche Products had chosen not to participate in the VPRS but the DHSS suspected that unacceptably high profits were being made at its expense from Valium and Librium, so it took the unprecedented step of referring the case through the Secretary of State for Trade and Industry to the Monopolies Commission. In February 1973 the Monopolies Commission reported that 'monopoly' conditions did prevail and recommended price cuts of 60 per cent for Librium and 75 per cent for Valium. Roche Products appealed against this and after a protracted legal battle the dispute was settled out of court in November 1975. Roche was required to join the VPRS and to repay part of the estimated £12 million excess profits. The balance was allowed to Roche to offset losses caused by inflation and exchange rate changes. From then on, prices for Valium and Librium were allowed to rise in accordance with the terms of the VPRS.

Hoffmann-La Roche is not necessarily representative of other pharmaceutical companies either in terms of its organisation or its relations with governments. The description of this case however reflects the problems that can arise when an unavoidable dependent relationship develops between the government and a sector of private industry. Although most pharmaceutical manufacturers would, in the case of the NHS, acknowledge the need for some government involvement in their affairs, they fundamentally criticise governments' accuracy in defining reasonable levels of profitability.[15]

Paramedical Staff

The work of the different types of paramedical staff is extremely varied, but as a whole it represents an identifiable and essential component in the whole programme of clinical care, without which medicine and nursing would be of limited effectiveness.

Many of the staff discussed in this section share the fact that their work is supervised directly or indirectly by doctors, and that most of them undergo training that is as long and thorough as nurses' training. Most of the occupations owe their development to the clinical and technical advances in medical science of the twentieth century. As medicine has become more sophisticated, specialisation within the profession has increased, and with it has come the need for specialist supporting staff to provide the necessary back-up services. There are a number of landmarks which should be mentioned before the individual professions are discussed. The first was in 1936, when the British Medical Association set up an independent Board of Registration of Medical Auxiliaries, incorporated under the Companies Act. Its object was to maintain and publish the National Register of Medical Auxiliary Services, listing those people who had satisfied the Board of their qualifications to practise. This arose because the doctors had become concerned that some of the techniques could involve risks if administered by untrained people. The result was that the professional organisations of dispensing opticians, dieticians, orthoptists, physiotherapists, speech therapists, chiropodists and radiographers became recognised by the Board, and their members were bound not to work except under the direction of a doctor, while the doctors undertook to refer patients only to duly qualified practitioners. This arrangement could not stop unqualified practitioners from working, since registration was entirely voluntary.

In this context, a committee was set up by the Minister of Health after the inception of the NHS, to consider 'the supply and demand training and qualifications of certain medical auxiliaries employed in in the NHS'. The result was the Cope report[16] which comprised separate analyses of the situation for almoners, chiropodists, dieticians, medical laboratory technicians, occupational therapists, physiotherapists and remedial gymnasts, radiographers and speech therapists. It recommended that statutory registration for medical auxiliaries working in the NHS should be necessary through separate registers. These registers and the recognition of approved training courses and examinations should be the responsibility of a single council with a number of constituent professional committees. Although these proposals were welcomed by the doctors and medical auxiliaries alike (but for different reasons), a long debate ensued between them over membership of the new bodies. In 1954, as an interim measure, regulations were introduced for the qualifications required for state registration of eight categories of staff by the NHS: chiropodists, dieticians, medical laboratory technicians, occupational therapists, physiotherapists, radiographers, remedial gymnasts and speech therapists.

Finally in 1960, the Professions Supplementary to Medicine Act was passed. This established the Council for Professions Supplementary to Medicine (CPSM), and seven Boards, one for each of the professions mentioned above, excluding speech therapists. The Boards were made legally responsible for the preparation and maintenance of registers, for prescribing qualifications required for state registration, and for approving entrance requirements, training syllabuses and training institutions. They can remove practitioners from the register for professional misconduct, and impose penalties for the improper use of the designation 'state registered'; they can also withdraw approval from training courses that fall below required standards. In 1966 the provisions of the Act were extended to include orthoptists. The Board of Registration of Medical Auxiliaries continued to provide for voluntary registration of chiropodists, orthoptists, dispensing opticians, operating theatre technicians, technicians in venereology, audiology technicians and certified ambulance personnel. The Council for Professions Supplementary to Medicine is itself composed of one member from each of the Boards, six nominees of the medical corporations and the GMC, four nominees of the Privy Council (including the Chairman) and five nominees, giving a total of twenty-three.

One further point to be made at this stage is that these paramedical and scientific occupations share problems of status and managerial authority in relation to other groups, particularly the doctors. It might be said that the move by the BMA to institute registration of medical auxiliaries was an attempt to exert control over other professions that it regarded as a threat rather than an asset. Equally, these professions probably welcomed registration since they saw it as an opportunity to expose charlatans and to close the ranks of truly qualified practitioners.[17] The wranglings over the constitutions of the boards recommended in the Cope report arose because the medical profession wanted to secure majority representation, but this did not eventually happen. The overall problem is that each of the occupations has to reconcile its desire for independent professional status with the inevitable fact that it serves the medical profession. They have to accept some degree of direction and control by the doctors, yet they regard themselves as competent specialists in their own right. Chapter 7 of the Grey Book[18] on the organisation of paramedical services, did not meet with the agreement of the professions concerned when it was published in 1972. The disagreements centred on this problem of their accountability to doctors, particularly in the predominantly hospital based professions. During the 1970s the debate continued. The Royal Commission had little to say on the matter of status, directing the comments to the need to review manpower and training needs of the professions. A DHSS circular in 1979[19] was inconclusive but the 1982 reorganisation re-opened the issue of status and accountability. Some professions such as speech therapy and chiropody had since 1974 been organised on an Area basis; the devolution of their services to Districts was seen as a loss of status. Most Districts had District heads of services although these became the objects of criticism in the post-*Patients First* discussions on the grounds that people who were trained to lay hands on patients were engaged in too much administration. Circular HC(80)8[20] left DHAs to decide how best to organise these professions in the future but warned against filling posts at District level unless there was adequate work to justify such a post. Managerially, accountability was split between the District Administrator and the District Medical Officer according to local agreement, and it is important to note that it was not seen as the automatic responsibility of the DMO or of a hospital consultant to supervise some of these professions.

The debate on professional autonomy seems likely to continue. In the therapeutic professions (physiotherapy, occupational therapy, dietetics, etc.) this causes little concern as their contribution to the therapeutic team is appreciated by medical staff. However doctors are much less happy at losing any further control of some of the technical professions such as laboratory technology or radiography.

Each profession will now be described. The relative numbers in practice are as given in Figure 29.

Figure 29 *Paramedical Staff* (March 1984)

Chiropody	5533
Dietetics	2088
Occupational Therapy	7126
Physiotherapy	17563
Remedial Gymnasts	603
Orthoptics	892
Speech Therapy	2278*
Clinical Psychology	1100

* September 1982

Chiropody

This is the treatment of superficial ailments of the feet, and the maintenance of the feet in good condition. In the eighteenth century chiropodists also cared for hands, but now they specialise in the treatment of existing deformities with appliances and special footwear, diagnosing and treating local infections, as well as preventive care, including the inspection of children's feet. Most chiropodists work in the community, holding clinics and making domiciliary visits. They work independently and do not require referral from a doctor, whereas those working in the hospitals work far more through referrals.

The Incorporated Society of Chiropodists was founded in 1912 to promote study and training and to improve services for poor people. In 1913 the London Foot Hospital was founded − the first specialist hospital of this kind. A number of other professional organisations grew up and in 1937 five of these were recognised by the Board of Registration of Medical Auxiliaries. They amalgamated to form the Society of Chiropodists in 1945, but there continued to be a range of bodies examining and registering chiropodists. The 1954 regulations laid down conditions for state registration and employment in the NHS, and the Chiropodists Board of the Council for Professions Supplementary to Medicine replaced these in 1963. In this year, it became the single body responsible for state registration, following a three year full-time course at an approved training centre. In 1975, about one third of all NHS treatments, including those done at patients' homes, were carried out by private chiropodists who received a fee from the NHS. The DHSS admits that chiropody services are inadequate, even for the priority groups − the elderly, the handicapped, expectant mothers, school children and some hospital patients. In 1977 it issued circular HC(77)9 which recommended various measures to the Area Health Authorities to enable them to make better use of their existing resources. Of particular importance was the suggestion that 'foot care assistants' could be employed to carry out simple treatments such as basic foot care and hygiene, for which the skills of the fully-trained chiropodist were not necessary.

Dietetics

A dietician applies knowledge of nutrients contained in food, the effect of preparation and cooking on them and their use by the body, to advise on suitable diets as part of the treatment of illness, as well as constructing diets for people with chronic disorders (e.g. diabetes, kidney disease). Most dieticians work in hospitals, in conjunction with the catering manager, and also follow up patients through out-patient clinics. In addition, there are some openings for them in the community services, for instance in advising mothers at ante-natal and post-natal clinics on the balanced diets required for their babies, and in the nutritional values of meals on wheels.

The first training schools for dieticians were established in the United States in the 1920s, and their students were trained nurses. In 1925 special diet kitchens were opened at one or two hospitals in London, Edinburgh and Glasgow, and they accepted students who had pure science or domestic science qualifications. In 1933 a special training course for dieticians was started at the King's College of Household and Social Science and the therapeutic work of these 'early' dieticians mostly involved the weighing and preparing of foods. Later, the development of drugs partly overtook the effect of dietetics in treatment of certain conditions. The British Dietetic Association was founded in 1936 and joined the voluntary registration scheme before the institution of requirements for state registration in 1954. Since 1963 the Dieticians Board of the Council for Professions Supplementary to Medicine has been the responsible regulating body.

In the reorganised NHS, dietetic services are managed on a District basis through the appointment of a District Dietician, who gives advice to the DMT and the DHA on the planning and provision of a nutrition and dietetic service. The District Dietician is accountable to the District Administrator for these management tasks while she and her colleagues work in a service-giving relationship to doctors.[21]

Occupational Therapy

This covers any work or recreation prescribed and guided by a doctor for the purpose of facilitating recovery from disease or injury. Patients are referred to the occupational therapist by a doctor, and most work is done in general and psychiatric hospitals and rehabilitation centres. There are some, though, who work in the community, in units for emotionally disturbed and autistic children, in work and day centres, and who make domiciliary visits. A number work in local authority social services departments, advising on adaptations and other requirements for the disabled. Occupational therapy has long had a place in mental hospitals, where it was provided by untrained craft workers until 1930 when the first training courses were started. The last war influenced its development through the need to provide for soldiers who were injured or shocked from combat.

The Association of Occupational Therapists was formed in 1936 and it registered occupational therapists who had passed the professional examinations after a prescribed three year course. After 1963, qualified practitioners became registered by the Occupational Therapists Board of the Council for Professions Supplementary to Medicine. The Halsbury report[22] noted that recruitment difficulties were accounted for by the fact that the NHS offered occupational therapists lower salaries than they could receive in local authority work.

Physiotherapy

Physiotherapy is the use of physical means to prevent and treat injury or disease, and to assist rehabilitation. People of all ages with a great variety of conditions can receive physiotherapy. The methods include therapeutic movement, electrotherapy, hydrotherapy, manipulation and massage. Most hospitals have departments treating outpatients and inpatients, and community work includes clinic sessions, work at rehabilitation centres and special schools for handicapped children. Treatment follows referral from a doctor and, as with many other state registered professions, physiotherapists undertake to treat only those who have been so referred.

The origins of physiotherapy started in a body called the Society of Trained Masseuses, founded in 1895. It was open to women only but in 1920 it became known as the Chartered Society of Massage and Medical Gymnastics and men were then admitted. The profession developed in scope and to reflect this the name was changed in 1943 to the Chartered Society of Physiotherapy. The society registered qualified practitioners, conducted examinations and approved training schools. After the Cope report and the 1960 Act, the Physiotherapists Board of the Council for Professions Supplementary to Medicine became the regulating body. The three year training courses of the Society are the only ones recognised for state registration.

Remedial Gymnastics

This profession is concerned with the treatment and rehabilitation of patients through active exercise. Special apparatus, games and exercises may be used, following medical diagnosis and referral, for a range of conditions including functional training in preparation for work and special work with mentally ill and handicapped patients. After the last war this more active type of physiotherapy was developed and training courses were set up.

The Society of Remedial Gymnasts issues a certificate after successful completion of a three year course, which is recognised by the Remedial Gymnasts Board of the Council for Professions Supplementary to Medicine.

The Remedial Professions as a Group

These three professions — occupational therapy, physiotherapy and remedial gymnastics — form a sub-group known as the remedial professions. Although they each have a distinct part to play, there are also some similarities and their work may sometimes overlap. In 1969 a government committee was set up (chaired by Professor Sir Ronald Tunbridge) to consider their interrelationships, since the professions felt dissatisfied with their pay, career prospects and professional status. The Committee's statement in 1972[23] recommended representation on advisory committees to the health authorities, adequate departmental establishments, better provision for aides (unqualified assistants), clerical staff and porters, integrated departments, re-employment of trained married women, and a review of the training syllabuses leading to an integration of the schools.

The professions were far from pleased with these points since they felt strongly about their independence and the lack of recognition. The Oddie report (Report of the Committee on Remedial Professions of the CPSM)[24] tried to press their case further but it was not until 1975 that they felt the problems had been acknowledged. A working party was set up by the Secretary of State to make urgent recommendations, and its report (the MacMillan report)[25] suggested that the professions of physiotherapy and remedial gymnastics should amalgamate, and in the long term the three should evolve into a single comprehensive profession; increased professional and managerial responsibility should rest with the practitioners; new career structures should be devised to reflect this; new methods of training, increased use and recognition of aides and recognition of the need for research should all be developed. A coordinating committee to deal with the implementation of these recommendations was set up in March 1975, and in particular to work out the details on some of the more complicated points such as the managerial relations between the professions, greater flexibility in the training, and the use of aides. Progress towards these aims has been slow. It seems unlikely that one profession will emerge from three although the future of remedial gymnastics is likely to be increasingly bound up with physiotherapy. Experiments with some joint training have not had much success, particularly given the degree status aspirations of the existing three year training schemes in physiotherapy and occupational therapy. However, the use of aides (physiotherapy) and helpers (occupational therapy) has developed with approved part-time training courses being set up in some Districts.

Orthoptics

This is the investigation of squints and other defects of binocular vision. Orthoptists work with medically qualified eye specialists and only treat patients referred to them by doctors. The majority of patients are children and most orthoptists are women. The British Orthoptic Council was founded in 1930 and runs a full-time two year course leading to a diploma. The Board of Registration of Medical Auxiliaries registered orthoptists until 1966, when the Orthoptists Board of the CPSM was set up to take this over.

Two other paramedical professions are concerned with therapy although they are not under the supervision of the CPSM. They are speech therapy and clinical psychology. A third profession, social work, whilst not paramedical, nevertheless provides support to medical and nursing staff.

Speech Therapy

This is the treatment of defects and disorders of the voice and speech. Originally, the work concentrated on stammering but after about 1912 hospital departments and local authority clinics began to be set up to offer treatment for the range of disorders. The 1944 Education Act obliged local education authorities to provide treatment for children with speech disorders, so the profession became split between those working in the education and health services (the ratio is about 3:1, education:health). There was a great demand for speech therapists as a result and the College of Speech Therapists was formed in 1945 to press for independent status of the practitioners. The profession has faced serious problems for some time: the small numbers of fully trained members; the fact that most of them give less than five years service; few senior posts make the career structure unattractive; research and preventive work has not developed; there is poor communication between the profession and medicine.

In 1972 the Quirk report (on speech therapy services) was published[26] and it contained proposals for reorganising and developing the profession so that it could cope with its expanding role in the NHS and the education service. It recommended that AHAs should be responsible for organising the practitioners in a suitable career structure and that training courses should be jointly arranged with universities so that the quality of the training might be enhanced. It also proposed a new central council to handle course assessment and registration of qualified practitioners and that the College of Speech Therapists should remain as a professional body only, its present examining role being taken on by the central council. The government approved the recommendations and in April 1974 issued guidance to AHAs on how they might begin to integrate their speech therapy services along these lines through the appointment of Area Speech Therapists.[27] It was acknowledged that the transformation of the profession would take some time. Since 1982 speech therapy has usually been organised on a District basis.

Clinical Psychology

The role of the clinical psychologist has become increasingly important. In mental illness clinical psychologists have a crucial role, not only in assessment but also in devising appropriate regimes of treatment. In mental handicap they formulate training plans for those mentally handicapped people who are being prepared to live in the community. They have a potential contribution to more clinical specialties and particularly family support, child health and rehabilitation. The Trethowan report (1977)[28] emphasised the professional autonomy of clinical psychologists, but felt that as they were used to working as part of a therapeutic team that would not lead to relationship problems. Clinical psychologists have to possess a first degree in psychology following which they undertake a further two years of specialist training.

Social Work

Social work has its roots in the almoner's department of pre-war hospitals which were particularly concerned with the financial status of patients, a matter of significance in voluntary hospitals which relied on contributions from patients as well as donations from the general public. From this came a general concern for the patients' circumstances so that social workers in hospital now have a particular responsibility for satisfactory discharge arrangements. In 1974 medical social workers ceased to be employed by health authorities and were transferred to local authority social services departments. This move was brought about by the Seebohm report (1968)[29] which recommended a single social work service with full professional status. Medical social workers, often more highly qualified than social workers coming from the fields of residential care or mental welfare, were reluctant to make the change. In the event most social service departments have maintained social workers in hospitals and honoured their specialism whilst enlarging their areas of concern.

Scientific and Technical Staff

The Zuckerman report (1968)[30] proposed a reorganisation of the scientific and technical services provided by medical laboratory technicians, some of the professions supplementary to medicine and others in the hospital service. The report included the following professions in its scheme as shown in Figure 30. The report recommended the creation of a National Hospital Scientific Council to advise the Ministers on the organisation of the hospital service, that might become one of the Standing Advisory Committees of the Central Health Services Council. Each Regional Hospital Board was to have an advisory committee, and at district general hospital level the report recommended a Division of Scientific Services to include medical and scientific staff involved in clinical biochemistry, computer science and statistics, genetics, haematology and blood transfusion, immunology, medical microbiology, morbid anatomy and histopathology, physics with biomedical engineering, nuclear medicine and physiological measurement. Four classes of staff were proposed; scientific officer, technical officer, technical assistant and technical aide, to reflect different degrees of responsibility and knowledge and to provide an improved career structure.

These recommendations did not survive and throughout the 1970s piecemeal alterations to the organisation of the services were made. Medical physics, a relatively new profession, developed with the encouragement of doctors but medical laboratory sciences were not given similar recognition and where some degree of autonomy was claimed serious conflict developed.

Figure 30 *Hospital Scientific Staff*

Biochemists
Physicists
Other scientific officers
Audiology technicians
Cardiology technicians
Darkroom technicians
Dental technicians
Electroencephalography technicians
Medical laboratory technicians
Medical physics technicians
Radiographers
Dieticians
Animal technicians
Artificial kidney technicians
Contact lens technicians
Electronics technicians
Glaucoma technicians
Heart and lung machine technicians
Respiratory function technicians
Surgical instrument curators
Surgical and orthopaedic appliance technicians and fitters

Source: Hospital Scientific and Technical Services, HMSO, 1969.

As can be seen from the list above these staff are somewhat loosely classified under one heading. They include some who have an extended training requirement (e.g. physicists), but also, others who may have practically no formal training (e.g. darkroom technicians). Three groups need special note.

Medical Laboratory Sciences

This group of staff is concerned with facilities for diagnosis and treatment of illness through examination of pathological specimens from outpatients and inpatients, and sent in from GPs' patients, under the supervision of consultant pathologists in the hospitals. The Pathological and Bacteriological Assistants' Association was founded in 1912 and in 1921 an examining council of the Pathological Society was set up to develop a system of certification. The Institute of Medical Laboratory Technology (now Sciences) was incorporated in 1942 as the single professional organisation. It registered qualified technicians who had worked in approved laboratories and attended part-time courses. The 1954 regulations for medical auxiliaries laid down the requisites for state registration and in 1963 the Medical Laboratory Technicians Board of the Council for Professions Supplementary to Medicine became the regulating body. Entrants to the profession need 'A' levels before proceeding to a Higher National Certificate (HNC) or, in three centres — Bristol, Birmingham and Coventry — the Higher National Diploma (HND). Twenty-five per cent of entrants now have degrees which entitles them to two years exemption from the three year qualifying requirement before being eligible for state registration as a Medical Laboratory Scientific Officer. Subsequent training leading to Fellowship is in one or more sub-specialties, such as biochemistry, haemotology, and by means of exams set by the Institute of Medical Laboratory Sciences.

Medical Physics

The origins of medical physics were in radiotherapy. With the increasing need to give expert support to doctors using technological equipment, an independent profession developed, becoming recognised in the founding of the Hospital Physicists Association (HPA) in 1943. Hospital physicists need a minimum qualification of a degree in physics, engineering or associated subject. The HPA have recently organised a two year in-service training scheme but advancement to the higher grades is unlikely without an MSc or PhD degree. The 1200 or so members of the HPA are not required to be registered but discussions are taking place on the best way of safeguarding professional standards.

Radiography

X-rays were discovered in 1895 and they are used to help diagnose illness and injury, and to provide treatment for certain malignant and other conditions. Until 1920, non-medical assistants were employed, but in that year the Society of Radiographers was formed to organise training courses and examinations and to register qualified practitioners. Both diagnostic and therapeutic radiographers work under the direction of doctors and there are standard protective and monitoring devices to ensure that they are not excessively exposed to radiation. Radiography is a hospital-based service.

In 1983 the training scheme was increased to three years of which the first part is common to both diagnostic and therapeutic radiography students. Schools of Radiography are attached to specific hospitals. After qualification radiographers are required to register with the Radiographers Board at the CPSM. In March 1984 there were 13,379 so registered. Changes in medical technology are having an effect on the content of radiographers' work and the more senior posts will usually specialise. Over 80 per cent of radiographers perform diagnostic work and the remainder therapeutic work.

Ancillary Staff

There are well over 400,000 patients in hospital on any one day in the year, who have the sheets on their beds provided by the laundry staff, who eat three meals cooked and served by the catering staff in wards cleaned by the domestic staff. Equipment and sterile dressings are provided by the supplies staff, while porters fetch and carry specimens and equipment and conduct patients around the hospital. In addition, certain staff live in the hospital, so some of the 'hotel' services are required for them. Most of the ancillary functions are not exclusive to the NHS and arise wherever meals and residential accommodation need to be provided. The community health services clearly require these services on a smaller scale since they are mostly concerned with non-residential care. Hostels and homes in the community are run by the social services departments unless they provide medically supervised care, in which case the ancillary staff would be employees of the District Health Authority.

In 1970 the DHSS issued advice aimed at improving the management of support services.[31] New posts of considerable seniority were set up which in 1974 were to become District Catering, Domestic and Linen Service Managers. By 1982, however, functional management (as it was called) had been discredited largely because of the tension between local unit or hospital administrators and the District functional managers endeavouring to supervise services from a distance.

A further change to ancillary services came in 1983 with the government's campaign for privatisation.[32] DHAs were directed to check the efficiency of their support services in the open market. When an outside contractor for domestic, catering or laundry work could provide a cheaper service than in-service staff, the employment of such staff was terminated and the outside contractors employed. Money thus saved could be used to benefit patients in other ways.

Works Staff

This group of staff includes architects, quantity surveyors, engineers, building supervisors, electricians, painters, carpenters, ground maintenance staff and labourers. They deal with the planning, construction and maintenance of the buildings, plant and grounds of the health service and, as with the ancillary staff, they are concentrated on the hospital side. The senior works staff based with the Regional Health Authorities hold professional qualifications such as those of the Royal Institute of British Architects, the Royal Institution of Quantity Surveyors and the various engineering institutions. Senior works staff of the districts have technical qualifications, but the pattern amongst them and the skilled and other works staff is to belong to a trade union rather than a professional organisation.

The stock of hospitals taken over by the NHS in 1948 included over 1,200 (45 per cent) that had been erected before 1891, and many were obsolete, poorly maintained, or in unsuitable locations. In the late 1950s, money began to be specially earmarked for the development of hospital building, and in 1962 the publication of *A Hospital Plan for England and Wales*[33] specified 90 new and 134 substantially remodelled hospitals to be started by 1970/71. It acknowledged the shortage of architects and engineers skilled in hospital planning, and in the same year the report of a study group investigating hospital engineering was published.[34] It recommended a number of steps to improve the training and quality of engineers, and suggested a minimum qualification requirement for employment in the NHS, as well as recognition of the group engineer as a chief officer. The Woodbine Parish report[35] published in 1970 made further recommendations for the improvement of building maintenance and the training of supervisory staff. When the Grey Book's scheme for works staff in the reorganised NHS was published, it met with opposition from the professions concerned. Revised guidance was issued in 1974[36] acknowledging some degree of autonomy for works staff such that responsibility was shared between senior works officers and administrators for the execution of building and maintenance. This specified the new posts and their management arrangements (particularly the Area and District works and building officers and engineers), their departmental organisation and degree of accountability to administrators. Nevertheless, because these functions constitute such a costly element in spending by authorities, the Department has always been concerned to monitor standards and local practices carefully, and it does this through a series of publications which give detailed advice and specifications about all aspects of health authorities' building, upgrading and maintenance work.[37] The Ceri Davies report (1983)[38] felt that works departments were too concerned with capital building schemes and with engineering plant at the expense of the wider issue of estate management. The report suggested a change of title from Works Officer to Estates Officer. Following the example of local authorities, health authorities may be tempted to review their direct labour works force and privatise significant parts of it.

Administrative and Clerical Staff

The Grey Book gave three reasons for employing administrators in the NHS: to manage institutional and support services, to provide administrative services, and to act as general coordinators. In practice this means that ambulances, laundry and central sterile supply, medical records, catering, portering and domestic services, supplies and personnel each have a manager who is responsible for the work of his department at District level (but not usually at Regional level, since institutional and support services are rarely organised there) to a senior administrator. Administrative services play a part in every aspect of the NHS and include secretarial support, management services and personnel management, public relations and legal advice for the range of staff and managers. General administrative coordination involves assisting different departments and professions to work cooperatively through multi-disciplinary teams and through informal methods, in the interests of providing integrated patient care. The senior administrative posts created by the reorganisation at each level, that were mentioned in earlier chapters, are a key element of the new structure because of their role in moderating the balance between the authority of the central Department and the delegated responsibility allotted to Regional and District Health Authorities and District Management Teams. A new element of managerial responsibility has been introduced, with specific methods for discharging it – namely, through monitoring and coordinating as well as directing the work of others. This role was emphasised in circular HC(80)8[39] where attention was drawn to the District Administrator's responsibility for ensuring that the DHA's policies and priorities are being implemented.

The early hospital administrators (called stewards in the local authority hospitals and house governor or secretary in the voluntary hospitals) were responsible to the chief medical officer or the governing body for the day-to-day business. With the introduction of the NHS in 1948, and the newly created authorities (Regional Hospital Boards, Hospital Management Committees and Boards of Governors) a new pattern of staffing was created, separating senior staff (e.g. secretary, assistant secretary, finance officer and supplies officer) from the junior grades (general, clerical and higher clerical). Two important reviews of administrative and clerical staffing were carried out, one in 1957 (the Noel Hall report)[40] and the other in 1963 (the Lycett Green report).[41] They promoted new gradings and salary scales, and improvements in recruitment and training. One result of the Lycett Green report was the setting up of the National Staff Committee and Regional Staff Committees to oversee the long-term development of administrative and clerical staff through more systematic and effective recruiting drives and improved management training for senior and first-line posts. The majority of the most senior administrators now are graduates and are expected to hold the diploma of the Institute of Health Service Administrators.

The 1974 reorganisation saw a substantial increase in the number of administrators. This was not only because of the additional tier of management; an increase in legislation, more specialisation in planning and personnel work particularly, and an unprecedented increase in industrial disputes all contributed to the need for more staff.

However, the growth of administrative staff has met with sharp criticism and moves to economise were set in motion in 1975. RHAs were asked to devise schemes for reducing management spending, and there has been a standstill in 'management costs' at the proportion of revenue which existed at 31 March 1976. By 1983, ministers were claiming in Parliament that £64 million had been saved as a result of the 1982 reorganisation, one of the reasons for which had been to reduce the size of the NHS bureaucracy.[42]

Notes

1. *Royal Commission on Doctors' and Dentists' Remuneration* (Chairman, Sir Harry Pilkington), HMSO, London, 1960 (Cmnd. 939).

2. Ministry of Health and Department of Health for Scotland. *Report of the Inter-Departmental Committee on the Remuneration of General Dental Practitioners* (Chairman, Sir Will Spens), HMSO, London, 1948 (Cmnd. 7402).

3. British Dental Association. *NHS Dental Treatment. What it Costs and How the Cost has Risen*, London, 1983.

4. *National Health Service Act, 1946*, HMSO, London, 1946, 9 & 10 Geo. 6 Ch 81, Section 41(4).

5. *Health Services and Public Health Act, 1968*, HMSO, London, 1968, Chapter 46.

6. Ministry of Health and Department of Health for Scotland. *Statutory Registration of Opticians*: Interdepartmental Report (Chairman, Lord Crook),

HMSO, London, 1952 (Cmnd. 8531).

7. Department of Health and Social Security. *Statement Specifying Fees and Charges for the Testing of Sight and the Supply or Repair of Glasses*, HMSO, London.

8. DHSS. *Health Service Development. Professional Advisory Machinery*, Para. 26, January 1982.

9. Department of Health and Social Security. *Report of the Inquiry into the Prescription Pricing Authority*, by R.I. Tricker, HMSO, London, 1977.

10. Ministry of Health. *Final Report of the Committee on the Cost of Prescribing* (Chairman, Sir Henry Hinchliffe), HMSO, London, 1959.

11. The reference to overseas prices actually favoured the UK industry since its prices in the home market were comparatively lower.

12. In at least one case, the supplies were found to fall short of expected standards.

13. *Report of the Committee of Enquiry into the Relationship of the Pharmaceutical Industry with the National Health Service 1965-1967* (Chairman, Lord Sainsbury), HMSO, London, 1967 (Cmnd. 3410).

14. It is the view of some observers (and notably those connected with the pharmaceutical industry) that the setting up of the Sainsbury Committee was a politically motivated act, and that the report itself reflected political rather than economic arguments.

15. See, for example: Runnymede Research Limited, *Competition, Risk and Profit in the Pharmaceutical Industry*. The Association of the British Pharmaceutical Industry, London, 1975.

16. Ministry of Health. Department of Health for Scotland. *Medical Auxiliaries*, Reports of the Committees (Chairman, Dr V. Zachary Cope), HMSO, London, 1950 (Cmnd. 8188).

17. The effect of making state registration a requirement of employment in the NHS is a valuable asset to these professions. It protects their name and educational standards, and also safeguards patients' interests.

18. Department of Health and Social Security. *Management Arrangements for the Reorganised National Health Service*, HMSO, London, 1972, p. 84.

19. DHSS Circular HC(79)19. *Management of the Remedial Professions in the NHS*, October 1979.

20. DHSS Circular HC(80)8. *Health Service Development. Structure and Management*, July 1980.

21. Department of Health and Social Security. *The Organisation of the Dietetic Service within the National Health Service*. Health Service Circular (Interim Series) HSC(IS)56, DHSS, London, July 1974.

22. Department of Health and Social Security. *Report of the Committee of Inquiry into the Pay and Related Conditions of Service of the Professions Supplementary to Medicine and Speech Therapists* (Chairman, Lord Halsbury), HMSO, London, 1975.

23. Department of Health and Social Security, Scottish Home and Health Department, Welsh Office. *Statement by the Committee on the Remedial Professions* (Chairman, Professor Sir Ronald Tunbridge), HMSO, London, 1972.

24. The Council for Professions Supplementary to Medicine. *Report and Recommendations of Remedial Professions Committee*, CSPM, London, 1970.

25. Department of Health and Social Security. *The Remedial Professions*, a report by a working party (Chairman, E.L. MacMillan), HMSO, London, 1973.

26. Department of Education and Science. *Speech Therapy Services*, Report of the Committee appointed by the Secretaries of State (Chairman, Professor Randolph Quirk), HMSO, London, 1972.

27. Department of Health and Social Security. *Speech Therapy Services:*

Interim Guidance, Health Service Circular (Interim Series), HSC(IS)22, DHSS, London, April 1974.

28. DHSS. *The Role of Psychologists in the Health Services* (Trethowan Report), HMSO, London, 1977.

29. *Report of the Committee on Local Authority and Allied Personal Social Services* (Seebohm Report), HMSO, London, 1965 (Cmnd. 3703).

30. Department of Health and Social Security, Scottish Home and Health Department. *Hospital Scientific and Technical Services*. Report of the Committee 1967–68 (Chairman, Sir Solly Zuckerman), HMSO, London, 1968.

31. DHSS Circular. Advance Letter A/L 4/70. Administrator and Clerical Staffs Whitley Council, May 1980.

32. DHSS Circular HC(83)18. *Competitive Tendering in the Provision of Domestic, Catering and Laundry Services*, 1983.

33. *A Hospital Plan for England and Wales*, HMSO, London, 1962 (Cmnd. 1604).

34. Ministry of Health, Scottish Home and Health Department. *Report of the Study Group on the Grading, Training and Qualifications of Hospital Engineers* (Chairman, Major-General Sir Leslie Tyler), HMSO, London, 1962.

35. Department of Health and Social Security. Scottish Home and Health Department. Welsh Office. *Hospital Building Maintenance:* Report of the Committee 1968–70 (Chairman, D. Woodbine Parish), HMSO, London, 1970.

36. Department of Health and Social Security. *Management Arrangements: Works Staff Organisation and Preparation of Substantive Schemes*, NHS Reorganisation Circular HRC(74)37, DHSS, London, October 1974.

37. *Hospital Building Notes. Hospital Technical Memoranda, Estmancode, Capricode, Data Sheets, Cost Allowance Guidance and Adapted Needleman Formula* are some of the titles. They are prepared and revised by the DHSS which distributes most of them; others are available through HMSO.

38. DHSS. *Underused and Surplus Property in the National Health Service*. Report of the Enquiry (Ceri Davies Report), HMSO, London, 1983.

39. Op. cit., para. 25.

40. Ministry of Health. *Report on the Grading Structure of Administrative and Clerical Staff* Sir Noel Hall, HMSO, London, 1957.

41. *Report of the Committee of Inquiry into the Recruitment, Training and Promotion of Administrative and Clerical Staff in the Hospital Service* (Chairman, Sir Stephen Lycett Green), HMSO, London, 1963.

42. House of Commons Parliamentary Debate. *Official Report (Hansard)*, p. 366, November 1983, HMSO, London, 1983.

11 PAY AND INDUSTRIAL RELATIONS

The setting of pay and conditions in the NHS has evolved through a system of collective bargaining. For many years this was entirely the responsibility of the Whitley Councils but by late 1983 about half the staff were relying on review bodies to agree their pay although these staff retained their links with the Whitley system for other conditions of service. This chapter starts by giving an account of the Whitley System and then discusses the criticisms made of it and the resulting changes. The second part of the chapter discusses industrial relations in the NHS, which many people believe have deteriorated over the last fifteen years.

Whitley Councils

The Whitley system originated in attempts to improve industrial relations during and after the First World War. J.H. Whitley (Deputy Speaker of the House of Commons) chaired a committee which recommended a three-tiered organisation for voluntary improvement in relations within industries, consisting of a national joint industrial council, district councils and local works committees, as well as a permanent arbitration body. A number of industries tried to implement such schemes, but many were not sustained, although a notable exception was the Civil Service, which operates through Whitley Councils to this day.

Before 1939 there was little application of the idea to health service staff, but during the Second World War, hospital labour was in short supply although urgently needed. The government intervened by fixing minimum wages for student nurses prepared to work in hospitals where the shortages were particularly acute, and by guaranteeing higher wages for assistant and trained nurses working in hospitals that were part of the War Emergency scheme. In 1943 the Rushcliffe (England and Wales)[1] and Guthrie (Scotland)[2] reports were published, recommending the wage rates for all ranks of hospital nurses and the committees remained in being to deal with revisions of their scales. In 1945, the Mowbray Committee[3] was set up to deal with domestic and similar hospital workers' pay, on a voluntary basis. It fixed national minimum rates and empowered provincial councils to fix higher local rates and to deal with local disputes. During the War, the National Joint Council for Local Authority Administrative, Professional Technical and Clerical Staff handled the negotiations for administrative and clerical staff of the local authority hospitals, while the British Hospitals Association and the Association of Hospital Officers (later the Institute of Health Service Administrators) held formal negotiations with the same groups of staff in the voluntary hospitals. In 1942, the Association of Clerks and Stewards of Mental Hospitals was wound up and members were advised to join the Association of Hospital Officers which then dealt with the administrative and clerical staffs' claims in the mental hospitals. In 1945, several of the paramedical professions arranged for joint negotiations with the employers through a voluntary committee, but the medical laboratory technicians (now scientific officers) remained outside this arrangement because their professional organisation did not want to jeopardise its status by entering into formally negotiated arrangements. The hospital owners therefore had to deal with those trade unions who had medical laboratory technicians as members.

The 1946 NHS Act laid down that all employees of non-teaching hospitals would work under the instruction of their Hospital Management Committee, although their employer at law was the Regional Hospital Board. Schedule 66 of the Act empowered the Minister of Health to make regulations about the qualifications, remuneration and conditions of service of any employee of the NHS. In 1947, the Ministry and the Secretary of State for Scotland drew up a scheme for a central joint body covering the whole service and for separate negotiating bodies for the main groups of staff.

The existing joint councils and committees naturally influenced the form of the new bodies, and all organisations with a claim to represent staff were appointed to the appropriate body. The result was one General Whitley Council and nine functional Whitley Councils. The functional councils determine pay and all those conditions of service requiring a national decision, affecting directly only those staff within its scope. The General Council's activities were, in practice, limited to matters of general application, e.g. determining travelling and sub-sistence allowances and the procedure for certain types of leave. The nine functional councils that were constituted were: Administrative and Clerical Staffs Council; Ancillary Staffs Council; Dental Whitley Council (Local Authorities); Medical and (Hospital) Dental Whitley Council; Nurses and Midwives Council; Optical Council; Pharmaceutical Council; Professional and Technical Staffs Council 'A'; Professional and

Technical Staffs Council 'B'; and, in addition, there was a Scottish Advisory Committee to ensure the Scottish interests were properly represented. The General Council also had a staff side and a management side, the staff representatives being members of the functional councils.

The Mowbray Committee became the Ancillary Staffs Council, the Rushcliffe and Guthrie Committees together became the Nurses and Midwives Council, and the staff members of the three bargaining bodies from the voluntary, local authority and mental hospitals amalgamated to form the Administrative and Clerical Staffs Council. For paramedical, scientific and technical staff there was unwillingness between the trade unions and professional associations to handle pay negotiations together, because these would involve the pay of professional workers who had paid for their own training as well as technicians who had served an apprenticeship. Many professional associations are registered as charities and this restricts their freedom to act as bodies representing their members' interests in formal wage negotiations. Trade unions are limited by the fact that they cannot force an unwilling employer to arbitration. The result was that two councils were set up for these staff which broadly (but not entirely) separate the trade unions and professional associations. On Professional and Technical Staffs Council 'A' staff who deal directly with patients were represented predominantly through professional organisations, and on Professional and Technical Staffs Council 'B' the rest (technicians, works staff, etc.) were represented mainly through trade unions. Separate councils were set up for those professional groups who could work as full-time employees in hospitals or for the local authorities, as well as being paid fees by the Executive Councils. Thus the Medical, Dental, Optical and Pharmaceutical Councils were set up.

By 1949, seven functional councils and the General Council were working, and in 1950 the Medical Council and the (Local Authority) Dental Council were set up. Hospital dental staff were brought within the scope of the Medical Council in 1962, and its name was changed to Medical and (Hospital) Dental Council. However the Doctors' and Dentists' Review Body took over the work of the functional Whitley Councils in relation to doctors and dentists from 1963 – see p. 182. Following the transfer of responsibility for ambulance services to the health authorities in 1974, a new Ambulancemen's Council was created.

On most functional councils staff organisations with relatively small membership claimed places alongside the major ones, and some trade unions with members in several branches of the health service gained places on more than one council. The composition of the management side reflects the curious position that the hospital authorities were in (as the health authorities now are) as a party to collective bargaining. Regional Hospital Boards and Boards of Governors were dependent on the government for all the money they spent. Clearly they could not agree or grant concessions to their staff unless the government was prepared to make money available, but, at the same time, the Ministry wanted to be involved in any discussions that might commit them to increased expenditure on wages. The management sides of the functional councils therefore consisted of officials from the Ministry of Health and Scottish Office, representatives from the Regional Hospital Boards, Hospital Management Committees and Boards of Governors, the Executive Councils (on Administrative and Clerical) and the local authorities (except on Administrative and Clerical). The relative under-representation of the RHBs, HMCs and BoGs in relation to the local authorities was perhaps surprising, but the hospital authorities were in no position to object. Following the reorganisation, representatives from the Regional and Area Health Authorities and the Scottish and Welsh authorities became members of the management sides, and local authority membership ceased. Health Authority membership increased after the McCarthy report *Making Whitley Work* (1976)[4] but decreased again in January 1984 in an attempt to develop a more streamlined and better informed management side.

The way the Whitley Councils work is for each side to meet separately to determine their attitudes and then as a joint body to discuss the issues together. Each side has a chairman and a secretary, the chair of the council alternating between the two sides from year to year, while the secretaries are joint secretaries of the full council. The staff side secretary is elected from staff representatives, and the management side secretary is an official of the DHSS. Regional and national appeals committees exist to hear the cases of employees who are aggrieved in any matter of their employment excluding disciplinary action or dismissal. Staff and management sides appoint equal numbers to the committees who jointly agree on a decision by a majority of both sides. The appeal can only be made by a trade union or staff association represented on a health service Whitley Council on behalf of the aggrieved employee. Staff also have access to industrial tribunals if they believe, for example, that they have been unfairly dismissed or discriminated against on the grounds of race or sex.

Why was the Whitley system criticised? First, it was very cumbersome. The large membership of each council, often over forty people, was not an efficient way of conducting business. The secretariat for the management side and the joint meeting was provided by the DHSS but frequently information required was not available and even routine committee business was not conducted in an efficient manner. Meetings were held in London and the expenses of members were considerable. Secondly, and more seriously, the Whitley system failed to produce coherence or consistency in pay bargaining even within councils and certainly not between councils. There was in effect no national Whitley strategy for NHS staff other than that contained within the government of the day's pay policy. Effective negotiation was often not possible because the management side were given little discretion by the government. On the staff side rivalry between trade unions made some settlements difficult to achieve. This was particularly evident when trying to transfer groups of staff from one council to another. For instance, the transfer of operating department assistants from the Ancillary Staffs Council to Professional and Technical 'B' took over five years to negotiate.

The limitations of the Whitley system led some groups of staff to seek better arrangements and in 1963 a permanent Review Body on Doctors' and Dentists' Remuneration was set up. Electricians and other craftsmen also achieved special direct negotiation arrangements with the setting up of the DHSS Craftsmen's Committee. Finally a Review Body for Nurses and Midwives and some professional and technical staff was set up in 1983 and the corresponding Whitley councils were left to deal with conditions of service only.

The McCarthy inquiry set up in April 1975 published its findings late the next year. The report did not propose a radically new system for NHS wage negotiations although most of the criticisms of the current arrangements were acknowledged. The report said that the Whitley Councils should be retained and strengthened, and that several important modifications should be made to ensure this. The major innovation suggested was that Regional Whitley Councils should be established as the forum for local negotiation, with the scope to fix specific details of settlements. As a consequence, the national Councils should negotiate more flexible agreements which leave room for interpretation and adaptation by the Regional Councils. In addition, the DHSS should loosen its grip over the management sides of the national Councils by only itself being concerned with the overall cost to government of settlements, and with any effects of agreements on major aspects of government policy. The health authorities should in turn take greater care to select experienced and committed representatives

Figure 31 *Trade Union and Professional Association Membership*

Total NHS staff	–	900,000 (all figures approximate)
of whom		600,000 belong to trade unions
COHSE, NALGO & NUPE together represent		500,000 staff
A further		200,000 staff belong to professional associations
leaving		100,000 staff belonging to neither type of body

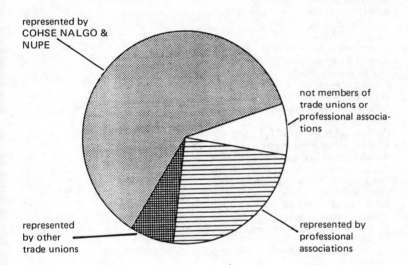

represented by
COHSE NALGO &
NUPE

not members of
trade unions or
professional associa-
tions

represented
by other
trade unions

represented by
professional
associations

TRADE UNIONS WITH LARGEST NHS STAFF MEMBERSHIP

COHSE	Confederation of Health Service Employees
NALGO	National & Local Government Officers Association
NUPE	National Union of Public Employees

OTHER UNIONS WITH NHS STAFF MEMBERS

ASTMS	Association of Scientific, Technical & Managerial Staffs
GMWU	General & Municipal Workers Union
NUGSAT	National Union of Gold, Silver & Allied Trades
TGWU	Transport & General Workers Union
UCATT	Union of Construction, Allied Trades & Technicians
USDAW	Union of Shop, Distributive & Allied Workers

PROFESSIONAL ASSOCIATIONS OF NHS STAFF
Administrative & Clerical
Assn of Hospital & Residential Care Officers
Assn of NHS Officers
Institute of Health Service Administrators

Society of Administrators of FPCs
Dental, Ophthalmic, Pharmaceutical
Assn of Dispensing Opticians
Assn of Optical Practitioners
Company Chemists Assn
Cooperative Union
Joint Committee of Ophthalmic Opticians
Pharmaceutical Council (Scotland)
Scottish National Ophthalmic Opticians
Socialist Medical Assn
Society of Opticians
Medical & Dental
British Dental Assn
British Medical Assn
Nursing & Midwifery
Assn of Nurse Administrators
Assn of Supervisors of Midwives
Health Visitors Assn
Royal College of Midwives
Royal College of Nursing
Scottish Assn of Nurse Administrators
Scottish Health Visitors
Professional & Technical
Assn of Clinical Biochemists
British Assn of Occupational Therapists
British Dietetic Assn
Chartered Society of Physiotherapists
Hospital Physicists Assn
Society of Chiropodists
Society of Radiographers
Society of Remedial Gymnasts

who were to be well briefed and required to report back.

Lord McCarthy's other main finding was the lack of coordination between organisations representing staff. He recommended a reduction in the total number through amalgamations, to produce more effective bodies, with agreed areas of recruitment in the NHS. He said that NHS employees should be consulted on all important management decisions and that his proposed improvements in the negotiating machinery should dovetail with improvements in the consultative procedures at national, regional and local levels. Although the government accepted all McCarthy's recommendations, only one improvement has actually been implemented — the management side members are now being better trained and briefed. However, other initiatives have been taken, such as new efforts to train managers in industrial relations techniques and discussions about improving local disputes procedures. But in its evidence to the Royal Commission on the National Health Service, ACAS (the Advisory, Conciliation and Arbitration Service, which has been called in to help resolve several disputes involving NHS workers) said 'In our view the NHS has reached the stage where it should review its industrial relations policies and practices. Unless effective remedies are introduced urgently, we see little prospect of avoiding continued deterioration.' This deterioration in industrial relations will be examined below.

The reform of the Whitley system made little progress. Discussions on an independent secretariat were prolonged but abortive. In 1983 a sub-group of RHA Chairmen assisted by NHS officers produced proposals aimed at simplifying the Whitley system by reducing the size of the management side. These proposals were warmly received by the Secretary of State and implemented on 1 January 1984. The new members spend much more time on Whitley affairs gaining a greater degree of expertise. But by this time, as we have seen, over half the staff had opted out of the Whitley system. Another significant event is the proposal in the Griffiths report that an NHS Personnel Director should be appointed. The role is not fully defined, but could imply that a radical review of pay bargaining in the NHS would be conducted.

Industrial Relations

It is commonly believed both within the NHS and outside that industrial relations have deteriorated within the service over the last fifteen years. Evidence of an increasing number of industrial disputes and of poor staff morale is cited. Whilst the former is quantifiable, the latter assumption needs careful handling. 'Morale' is a vague term, casually used. Many patients will be able to testify to the excellent spirit amongst staff in whose care they have been, although others will have witnessed staff shortages and insensitivity to patients' needs. Any large organisation faces problems of work distribution and worker motivation, so it is important to draw attention to those issues which have been particularly significant for the NHS and its staff.

The NHS is sometimes depicted in its early days as a happy family where everyone knew their place and all worked as a team. The break-up of the family is usually held to be the fault of ancillary staff, but the situation is rather more complicated than that; various events led to a change in the industrial climate. In the first twenty years of the NHS trade union membership was increasing. Over the last twenty years the Confederation of Health Service Employees (COHSE), a union with exclusively health service membership, has expanded from 30,000 to 200,000 members. The rather paternalistic management style began to change and a more realistic relationship developed between groups of staff, recognising the contribution each one had to make, but placing no group in a subservient relationship to another. But there were other factors. By the mid-1960s staff attitudes had changed to the point where they could contemplate industrial action to pursue their interests. In 1965 general practitioners, increasingly frustrated at the lack of material recognition, threatened mass resignations from the NHS. Following this in 1969 the Royal College of Nursing conducted a spirited campaign under the slogan 'Raise the Roof' through which they succeeded in obtaining a 22 per cent wage rise. But in the winter of 1973 ancillary staff completely' withdrew their labour in many places and took action which had a direct and damaging effect on patient care. Despite the bitterness this dispute caused, the nurses were again campaigning in 1974, openly stating that they could not promise to safeguard patient care if the government refused to listen. Both consultant and junior hospital doctors took action in 1975 over their pay, limiting the work they were prepared to do with a corresponding increase in waiting lists. The 1979 'winter of discontent'[5] ancillary dispute was if anything worse than the 1973 dispute except that hospital managers having faced the unthinkable that year, were now much more prepared to deal with the emergency and less likely to concede points. Throughout the 1970s, ambulancemen had taken sporadic action, some involving withdrawal of labour. The reasons for this increase in militancy are complex, but three broad causes were government policy, the problem of pay relativities, and an increase in employment legislation.

First, government policy. The 1974 Labour government was ideologically opposed to the continuation of private practice in general and private beds in NHS hospitals in particular. These had been a compromise in the negotiations with doctors over the setting up of the NHS in 1946. There were about 4,500 private beds within NHS hospitals which were seen as an anachronism in a service where medical need was the fundamental criterion for admission. Members of NUPE (the National Union of Public Employees, which represents many NHS workers) took up the matter and tried to close down private beds in NHS hospitals by refusing to service them. Medical staff retaliated and by 1976 only the setting up of the Health Services Board[6] broke the deadlock. The Board's task was to phase out private beds in a manner agreeable to both sides. The members of the board duly reflected the spirit of compromise with half from the medical profession and half from trades unions and people sympathetic to their views. The case illustrates how industrial relations within the NHS were affected, leaving the health authorities themselves powerless to remedy the cause of the dispute.

A second case required health authorities to do more than cope with the consequences of industrial action; they were required to enact the government's will. In 1983 the government instructed health authorities to test the efficiency of their support services in the open market. The DHSS prepared specimen tender documents and directives ensured that DHAs did not write specifications favouring themselves. Indeed, by not allowing DHAs to specify that all contractors should prepare their quotations on the basis that staff should be paid Whitley Council rates, the DHSS specifically put in-house tenders at a disadvantage. Industrial action was made less likely following the implementation of this policy because ancillary staff were cowed by the prospect of unemployment.

Pay relativities have been the root of much industrial unrest in the NHS in recent years. It has already been shown how GPs and nurses threatened action when their pay negotiations seemed to be failing. The problem has affected all NHS staff in turn and various attempts have been made to make these negotiations less volatile by introducing some guiding principles. One of these was to leave room for local negot- iation. In 1968 the National Board for Prices and Incomes produced a report (Number 29)[7] on manual workers in the NHS, local authorities, and the gas and water supply industries. The incomes of these workers were relatively very low, but so was their productivity. What way could be found to improve the productivity without necessarily increasing the public authority's wage bill? Incentive bonus schemes were suggested to meet this need. These productivity schemes had been common in many industries, but had not been tried in the NHS before. Ancillary staff were offered the opportunity for a full work-studied scheme, and while they were waiting for that could be given a bonus of up to 10 per cent of their basic earnings on an agreed specification of work, providing the new productivity levels were self-financing. This could in effect only be done by losing staff. Bonus schemes were also introduced for works staff in the early 1970s. Bonus schemes remain although they have provided a fertile ground for disputes. In some respects they have made matters worse in that relativities have been distorted so that shift workers earning bonus payments have been able to get substant- ially more than their own supervisors. Similarly, untrained ancillary staff have been able to earn more than trained staff such as nurses. The negotiation of bonus schemes has required better local union

organisation and the number of shop stewards has increased. With this
has come an increased demand for facilities to conduct union affairs
such as time off and office space. These demands themselves have sometimes led to friction with management.

Another way of endeavouring to meet the relativities problem was
to bring in an outside committee to conduct an objective review.
Despite the substantial rise in pay in 1970, the rapid rise in inflation
that followed again left nurses badly off in relative terms. Towards the
end of 1974 Lord Halsbury headed a committee of six which was
appointed by the Secretary of State to investigate the pay of nurses
and midwives and also to inquire into the pay and conditions of service
for the eight paramedical professions that have been discussed in
Chapter 10. Their report was published early in 1975,[8] and it gave these
staff substantial pay increases. Traditionally, their pay has been linked
to nurses' pay – there are some similarities, since they share the same
employer and places of work, and they are (except for chiropody and
remedial gymnastics) predominantly women's professions in which
many work on a part-time basis. Halsbury found that no job evaluations
comparing the training and skills required for each of the professions
had been carried out, and he strongly recommended that this should
be done. He noted that substantial staffing shortages existed for most
of them in relation to NHS work, and suggested more full-time working
should be encouraged, since the actual numbers of individuals with
state registration indicated a potentially larger workforce. He justified
the large awards (made in the context of a statutory incomes policy) by
saying that they were ' . . . no more than have been due to these professions in recognition of their responsibilities and bearing in mind the
critical manpower shortages'. The effect of the awards was to improve
recruitment into these professions considerably. Staff shortages are less
than they were and in radiography, for example, sufficient staff can
now be employed.

Despite Halsbury, the problem of comparability would not go away.
In March 1979 the Prime Minister set up the Standing Commission on
Pay Comparability under Professor Clegg[9] to take a larger look at
comparability across a wide range of workers including, in the NHS,
ancillary staff, nurses, midwives and professions supplementary to
medicine and ambulancemen. The results of this exercise pleased
neither the staff who had expected more of it nor the government who
had hoped for less. Another attempt at comparability was undertaken
by Speakman[10] who examined the relative salaries of chief officers
without finding an acceptable formula. On a wider basis the Megaw

report[11] on civil service pay in 1982 tried to settle the dilemma of collective bargaining within government restraints. In the past, civil service pay had been a yardstick for setting the level of pay awards for NHS administrative and clerical staff, but from 1981 onwards this ceased. Megaw proposed that after a careful review of factors such as private sector pay rates, labour supply, needs of the service, efficiency, and the money available it should be possible to provide room for bargaining within upper and lower limits. But by 1984 these recommendations had made little progress in the civil service or in the wider field of public sector pay negotiations.

The third factor influencing industrial relations was the new employment legislation passed since 1970. Before that time the NHS had not employed specialist personnel officers, but thereafter local personnel specialists became essential for a District. The Health and Safety at Work Act 1974 requires all employers to take a much more rigorous look at the safety of their working environment. Certain parts of a hospital such as the laboratories, mortuaries and operating theatres could even be closed down if found to be unsafe by the Health and Safety Executive inspectors. In addition, health authorities were advised to set up health and safety committees to introduce or improve proper accident and untoward incident report systems. This went a great deal further than the previous requirements of the Factory Acts and the Offices Shops and Railway Premises Act. Disagreements over levels of safety have led to disputes between staff and management.

Much employment legislation has been introduced in recent years aimed at enhancing and safeguarding the rights of employees. Although some of it has been repealed by later governments, the acknowledgement of the need for effective representation of staff has remained. Health authorities are required to give reasonable facilities for trade union members and their shop stewards (negotiating what is 'reasonable' has, however proved far from straightforward). In the case of intractable disputes between a group of trade union members and management, the Advisory Conciliation and Arbitration Service (ACAS) can be brought in. ACAS was set up by the Trade Union and Labour Relations Act 1974, and it has survived various changes in legislation. But it has not always been particularly successful in achieving reconciliation in major, nationwide NHS disputes, partly because, as has been seen, local management have been constrained by government policy and instructions and have therefore been unable to negotiate freely.

It is not easy to see how industrial relations in the NHS will develop.

The Employment Act 1982 has limited trade unions' powers in industrial disputes principally by ruling secondary picketing illegal. NHS ancillary staff are anxious about the insecurity of their employment and whilst this anxiety remains it seems that industrial action will probably be limited. The power of the ancillary trade unions depends on their membership which could be substantially eroded by privatisation. But in 1984 many of the deep-seated problems remain. There is no coherent strategy on relativities and each pay award tends to be an attempt by one group to leap-frog another. The Whitley Council system is subject to substantial overhaul and the new nurses and midwives review body as yet unproven. More local negotiations on pay are favoured by some, but this might be inflationary as each District tried to offer better terms than its neighbours. The NHS cannot be exempt from the pay bargaining struggles facing all industries; even so, guidelines for the orderly conduct of these negotiations seem almost as remote as ever after thirty years.

Notes

1. Nurses' Salaries Committee. First Report. *Salaries and Emoluments of Female Nurses in Hospitals* (Chairman, Lord Rushcliffe), HMSO, London, 1943 (Cmnd. 6424).
2. Scottish Nurses' Salaries Committee. *Interim Report* (Chairman, Professor T.M. Taylor, later, Lord Guthrie), HMSO, London, 1943 (Cmnd. 6425).
3. National Joint Council for Staffs of Hospitals and Allied Institutions in England and Wales (Chairman, Sir George Mowbray).
4. DHSS. *Making Whitley Work* (McCarthy Report), London, 1976.
5. Several people claim the credit for this nickname including the General Secretary of NUPE, Rodney Bickerstaffe. The quotation comes from the opening lines of Shakespeare's Richard III 'Now is the winter of our discontent Made glorious summer . . .' The second half of the line seemed scarcely appropriate given that the ancillary staff did not get what they wanted.
6. The Health Services Board was set up under the Health Services Act 1976. It was dissolved by the Health Services Act 1980. More recently (1984) members of the private health care sector have regretted its loss on the grounds that it might help legitimate the relationship between public and private health care provision.
7. National Board for Prices and Incomes. Report No. 29. *The Pay and Conditions of Manual Workers in Local Authorities, the National Health Service, Gas and Water Supply*, HMSO, London, 1968.
8. DHSS. *Report of the Committee of Inquiry into Pay and Related Conditions of Service of Nurses and Midwives* (Halsbury Report), HMSO, London, 1974.
9. Standing Commission on Pay Comparability. Reports 1. Local Authority and University Manual Workers; NHS Ancillary Staffs; and Ambulanceman (Cmnd. 7641), HMSO, 1979. 3. Nurses and Midwives (Cmnd. 7795), HMSO, 1960. 4. Professions Supplementary to Medicine (Cmnd. 7850), HMSO, 1980.
10. *Review of Top Posts in the National Health Service.* A report to the Nurses

and Midwives, Administrative and Clerical and Professional and Technical (B) Whitley Councils. Prepared by A.J. Speakman, June 1971.

11. *Inquiry into Civil Service Pay*: a report of the enquiry into the principles and the system by which the remuneration of the non-industrial Civil Service should be determined (Megaw Report), HMSO, London, 1982 (Cmnd. 8590).

12 THE PUBLIC AND THE NATIONAL HEALTH SERVICE

This chapter is concerned with a range of issues that illustrate the relationship between ordinary people and the health services that are provided for them by the State. In the first section, statutory and other arrangements that relate directly to the public rather than to people who have become patients are discussed. The next section goes on to consider selected health care issues on which sections of the public have expressed their view, particularly in criticism of prevailing NHS policy.

Community Health Councils

Community Health Councils (CHCs), an innovation of the 1974 NHS reorganisation, are bodies whose broad task is to represent the views of local users of the health services to the health authorities. The idea of setting them up arose principally because it was felt that health service users had exerted too little influence on the provision and planning of services in an organisation that had become dominated by professionals. In the past, the tasks of managing the provision of services and monitoring their quality had been combined. Some members of the old hospital authorities and the former local authority health committees were specifically meant to represent the lay view, but their influence was felt to have been limited. On the new AHAs the lay members were appointed to shoulder managerial responsibilities, and the emphasis was to separate this from the responsibility for representing consumers' views. CHCs remained after the 1982 reorganisation. There is a CHC for each health district. They provide for over 6,000 people to play an active part within the health service as members of statutory bodies for expressing consumer opinion, quite separate from the health authorities which take care of the day-to-day running of the services.

CHC membership has been worked out principally on the basis of the resident district population, and ranges from 18 in the smallest to 24 in the largest. Half the members are nominated by the local authorities, one third by voluntary organisations and the remaining one sixth by the regional health authorities. RHAs have the job of officially appointing all the nominees, normally for a period of four years, and half the members retire every two years (although they are eligible for re-appointment). A limited number of people can also be coopted. Generally, each CHC has two full-time staff – the Secretary and his or her assistant – who work from offices chosen by the CHC. In some cases CHCs have obtained shop front accommodation while others work from offices which may be rented from the health or local authorities. The money to pay staff salaries, office costs and all other expenses is made available by the Regional Health Authorities on the basis of agreed budgets. The CHCs' staff are employees of the Regional Health Authorities and training opportunities for them and the members are arranged by the RHAs.

Circular HRC(74)4 issued by the DHSS outlined the organisation of CHCs and some of the subjects they might direct their attention towards, but it did not specify exactly what their role should be. In circular HC(81)5, which was able to draw on the experience of the first seven years of CHCs, the Secretary of State saw CHCs as 'local bodies representing the interests of their local population'. CHCs initially had to concentrate on becoming informed about the health care needs of the population and the degree to which local provision met this. They also had to develop working relationships with District Management Teams (Area Management Teams in single-District areas) and other officers and staff of the Area Health Authority, and to devise ways of putting their own views across. Community Health Councils still face a considerable difficulty in making their existence known to local people. To the majority of the population, questions of administration and planning in an organisation as extensive as the NHS are not interesting. Individuals tend to have views about 'illness' rather than 'health', and they tend to find it difficult to consider questions which extend beyond their own personal experience. This is not a criticism but a reflection of the very low priority which governments and authorities have given to explaining issues of policy and administration in a clear and honest way. Newspapers, radio and television are the principal sources of information about all aspects of national life for most people, and these are quite inadequate on the whole to enable people to develop a considered view of complex problems. So CHCs are faced with the task of providing a certain amount of information to interest the public and activate its awareness. Public meetings, advertisements, exhibitions as well as contact with many local groups and press briefings are some of the ways to do this. Through members' own contacts with voluntary organisations and the local authorities, the work of the CHC can be further explained and developed, but this all requires time and effort which may be in short supply. CHC members give their time voluntarily in addition to their other commitments, so the degree to which CHCs can become known and hence reflect the needs of local people is very dependent on the determination of the members and the staff.

The meetings of CHCs are open for members of the public to attend (as are those of the RHAs and DHAs) who may be given the opportunity to speak. People can also call at the CHC office for help and advice. If they have complaints about the NHS the CHC can explain how to make best use of the official channels and procedures. Although it is not the responsibility of CHCs to judge or investigate individual complaints, by playing an active part they can support people through what may be complex and bewildering encounters with the NHS administration and they can comment constructively on areas of complaint to the health authorities. In terms of their overall influence in the NHS it may appear that CHCs are relatively powerless – they certainly have no managerial responsibility for the provision of any services. But they do have the right to ask for and receive information from the administration; they have the right to send one of their members to DHA meetings; they have the right to visit NHS premises; they have the right to be consulted about development plans and to play a part in the annual planning cycle; consultation with them on hospital closures and substantial changes of use is obligatory; they can give evidence to official committees; they can enlist the support of MPs; and, above all, they can use the press to articulate their views forcibly.

Most CHCs have divided into working groups which each concentrate on a defined sector of health care by meeting regularly to consider information, conduct investigations, make visits and reports. CHCs also have to prepare an annual report to the RHA and there is a statutory annual public meeting with the DHA. In relation to the family practitioner services, CHCs have more limited official powers. They only have observers at the meetings of FPCs which permit this and they do not have automatic access to GPs' surgeries. As a result, many councils have found it advantageous to make their own informal contacts with doctors and the Local Medical Committee in order to establish an atmosphere of mutual respect and to improve the exchange of information. In contrast, a growing number of CHCs is being invited to send observers to the meetings of joint consultative committees; observer status or full membership of District planning teams is also increasingly common.

In May 1974 the Secretary of State issued a consultative paper called *Democracy in the NHS*[1] which put forward ways in which the government was prepared to strengthen the principle of delegated authority in the NHS. With reference to CHCs, the two main suggestions were that two members should be appointed to the AHA, and that a representative body should be created, to advise and assist CHCs, with a budget drawn from central funds. The paper announced firm decisions to allow the posts of CHC secretaries to be filled by open competition (instead of being restricted to within the NHS); to oblige DMTs to send a spokesman to CHC meetings when invited, to answer questions in open session; to include CHCs among the bodies consulted by RHAs, before making appointments to the AHAs; to make NHS employees and family practitioners eligible for CHC membership and to give CHCs a key role concerning hospital closures. CHCs, health authorities and other interested bodies were asked to submit their views on the paper's tentative proposals to the DHSS. In July 1975 the Secretary of State announced that in the light of these representations she had decided to allow each CHC to send one member to attend AHA meetings with the right to speak but not to vote. In 1976, circular HC(76)25 was issued by the DHSS amending the advice about appointing CHC members. It indicated that RHAs should include a trades council representative and a disabled person amongst its own nominees, and pointed out that all members of CHCs should be '. . . prepared to devote a considerable amount of time and energy to their Council's work. It is important that appointing bodies should take account of this, and confirm with prospective members that they can undertake the necessary duties before putting forward nominations'.

By the end of the 1970s there was a feeling that CHCs were not worth their annual level of expenditure, small though that was. This attitude may have arisen both as a result of too much CHC activity and too little. In a few cases, notably inner city areas, some CHCs had spearheaded an attack on government policy and had disrupted AHA meetings. But in many other areas the CHCs were relatively ineffectual, duplicating work largely done by AHA members themselves. The Royal Commission unequivocally supported the continuation of CHCs but *Patients First* was less sure and committed the government only to a further review. In the event, circular HC(80)8[2] announced that CHCs would continue for the time being and this was followed by a more detailed circular HC(81)15[3] revising membership numbers to make most CHCs smaller and clarifying other matters concerning the role of the CHC, and the method of appointing members. Ministerial statements

since have continued to support CHCs although not always with particular enthusiasm so that their long term future remains a matter for
debate.

Why should this be so? The original concept was to separate management from consumer representation. Since the 1982 reorganisation
with smaller and more local DHAs, members of these authorities do not
see these two functions as being so clearly differentiated. Before 1982
DMTs could use their local CHC to put pressure on the AHAs but this
no longer applies. In many places CHCs have not been very successful
in making their presence felt partly because, being made up of many
separate representative interests, it has been difficult to formulate a
clear point of view, particularly one which may be critical of government policy. Even hospital closures have been difficult for CHCs to
fight, conscious as they have to be that they will be expected to suggest
alternatives if their opinion is to be considered seriously. Finally CHCs
are reliant on DHAs and their staff for information and this tends to
reduce their power to do much more than give a second opinion on
plans.

The idea of a national body for CHCs was discussed for some time
until a meeting of CHC representatives decided in November 1976 to
proceed with its establishment. The first Annual General Meeting
of the Association of Community Health Councils for England and
Wales was held in June 1977, attended by representatives of more
than 70 per cent of CHCs who had decided to join. At the request
of the DHSS in 1975 a national information service for CHCs, including a regular publication called *CHC News*, was set up and spon-
sored by the King's Fund. This proved to be successful and in
1976 the DHSS assumed responsibility for its costs. The withdrawal
of financial support caused the end of publication in June
1984.

The reorganisation of the NHS and hence the creation of CHCs
occurred at a turning point in the history of health service provision.
Continued growth and expansion was for the first time seriously in
doubt, and the public expenditure cuts of successive governments in the
1970s had a significant effect on the NHS. CHCs were therefore not in
a position to expect demands for increased overall spending to be met,
but they were in a position to pioneer attempts to encourage shifts
in spending, particularly away from the hospital services towards the
community services. Despite the reservations outlined above they are,
through their knowledge of the way in NHS works, and through their
involvement in the planning cycle, potentially able to promote the

more effective use of limited resources, particularly in relation to the needs of the local community.

Complaints Procedures

CHCs are also in a position to help the public to make effective use of the official complaints procedures, which can seem bewildering to many people. Formal complaints about hospital services are handled by the District Administrator responsible for the hospital in question According to DHSS circular HM(66)15, informal complaints are usually dealt with on the spot by the head of the department, while any action following investigation of the complaint has to be agreed by the head of the hospital department involved. In both cases the complainant has to be informed of the outcome and told that he can pursue his complaint with higher authorities if he remains dissatisfied. The Davies report on hospital complaints procedure, which was published in 1973,[4] recommended several innovations including a detailed code of practice and the establishment of investigating panels. These panels would be quasi-legal bodies which would deal with serious complaints that could otherwise be taken to court. The report also prescribed a strong role for CHCs both in helping and advising people on how to make the best use of the procedure, and in commenting directly to the health authorities on issues that the CHCs considered potential areas of complaint. The government welcomed the report, but lengthy consultations lasted until 1976 when it was announced that a uniform code of practice would be implemented for hospital and community (but not family practitioner) services. Opposition to the proposed investigating panels delayed a positive decision so this point was referred to the Select Committee on the Parliamentary Commissioner for Administration, for further consideration. After further consultation, circular HC(81)5 was issued which gave expanded guidance for the procedures for handling hospital complaints. But it also introduced a major addition by setting up a procedure for dealing with complaints involving clinical judgement. This had always been a problem. Patients and their relatives dissatisfied with the answer to their complaints about clinical treatment had had only two alternatives – to accept the explanations, however inadequate, or to go to law. The new procedure, negotiated with considerable difficulty with the BMA, set out three stages. Stage one is the same as for any complaint investigation. The matter is drawn to the attention of the consultant (consultants are responsible for the actions of their juniors) and to the health authority's administrators. If the answer is unsatisfactory to the complainant, he or she then renews the complaint and asks for the Regional Medical Officer (RMO) to be involved. An informal reconciliation is attempted but if this fails the matter then passes to the third stage with the setting up of an independent professional review panel. Doctors sitting on this panel are paid £40 a day.

The new procedure was set up in September 1981 and after sixteen months a report was presented to the Sectretary of State[5] who concluded that the new arrangements were working well. RMOs had considered 184 cases and set up a review for sixty-three of them. Some complaints had been rejected because it was felt the complainant was using the procedure to obtain further evidence for litigation. Overall the procedure was welcomed, as it had dealt more satisfactorily with complaints arising from diagnosis and treatment (said to be about 43 per cent of all complaints). It should perhaps be added that the total number of complaints is very small given the millions of patient contacts each year.

In the case of complaints made against GPs, general dental practitioners, opticians and pharmacists providing NHS services, the complaint has to be made in writing to the family practitioner services administrator, normally within eight weeks of the event which gave rise to it. It has to allege a breach in the practitioner's terms of service: i.e. his contract with the FPC. The administrator initially tries to settle informally all those complaints that are relatively minor with the complainant, but if it is a more serious matter, he refers it to one of the Service Committees of the FPC. These are small bodies appointed by the FPC with professional and lay members, who hear the complaint and give the complainant and the practitioner the opportunity to present their cases and call witnesses. The Service Committee's decision can be appealed against by either party if it is adverse to them, in which case the Secretary of State can arrange for a small committee to consider the case again, sometimes with an oral hearing, both parties having the right to be legally represented. Various penalties can be imposed on a practitioner who is found to have breached his terms of service, and can involve a warning or a withholding of remuneration. In exceptional cases a practitioner can be referred by the FPC to the National Health Service Tribunal. This body has the power to remove a person from the FPC's list if continued inclusion would 'be prejudicial to the efficiency of the services'. The practitioner then has the right to appeal to the Secretary of State who may confirm or revoke the

Tribunal's decision. This procedure is distinct from the professions' own disciplinary powers to erase the name of a practitioner from the professional register and hence to disqualify that person from practising at all. A practitioner who has had his name removed from an FPC list by a decision of the NHS Tribunal is still free to practise privately or as a salaried employee of the NHS.

All these arrangements for investigating complaints are governed by the *Service Committees and Tribunal Regulations 1974* (as amended by Statutory Instrument 1974 No. 907) and the Council on Tribunals has suggested a number of improvements to them. In 1976 the DHSS initiated a review and invited interested parties to submit views on those suggestions and on any other improvements. In particular, the Council on Tribunals said that the Service Committee procedure could be criticised for being insufficiently independent since the FPC is responsible both for providing services and for deciding whether a complaint about them is justified. The machinery for hearing complaints rests entirely with the administering authorities and the professions which are the parties to the contractual arrangements. Furthermore, at Service Committee hearings, both parties can be assisted by a person of their choice provided that person is not a 'paid advocate'. The position of CHC secretaries as active helpers to patients under the regulations has led to some controversy, and the Council on Tribunals suggested that the term 'paid advocate' should be clarified in order to resolve the position of MPs, paid officials of trade unions and professional associations and CHCs. In 1978 the DHSS issued proposals for improving the procedures. These covered extension of the informal procedure, service committee chairmen to be drawn from a panel of legally-qualified people, changes in membership, role of the administrator, representation of parties by unpaid advocates, access to medical records, time limits, oral complaints and other points.

A further channel for the consideration of complaints was created by the appointment of the Health Service Commissioner under the 1973 Act. The Commissioner took up office on 1 October 1973 and is empowered to investigate complaints received directly from members of the public concerning failures in provision of services or incidents of maladministration by the health authorities in England, Wales and Scotland. These mainly concern grievances about the treatment and care of patients and the failures in communication between patients and the hospital staff. Specific examples quoted in the Commission's reports include complaints about the length of time patients have had to wait for hospital treatment, the repeated postponement of a major operation, and the performing of an operation without a patient's consent. The Health Service Commissioner is specifically excluded from investigating actions taken solely in consequence of the exercise of clinical judgement, personnel matters or any action taken by a person providing general medical, dental, pharmaceutical or ophthalmic services for which the FPC is responsible. Health authorities may also refer matters to him if they have been unable to resolve them satisfactorily. The Commissioner is based in London and has a small staff of civil servants and staff seconded from NHS work. There are also investigating units in Cardiff and Edinburgh, and thirteen members of the medical profession are available to give him advice in deciding whether a particular complaint from a patient involves clinical judgement. During his first eighteen month's work, the Commissioner received 973 complaints, 57 per cent of which had to be rejected as outside his jurisdiction (mainly because the body complained against had not been given the opportunity to consider the complaint first – this step being required by the Act before the Commissioner can take up the complaint). In the first ten years 6,824 complaints were received. Of these 4,458 were rejected, 993 referred back to the complainant and 1,178 investigated and reported on.

The Work of Voluntary Organisations

As the historical summaries in earlier chapters have shown, many of the existing health services have their origins in the work of volunteers and voluntary organisations – outstanding examples are the voluntary hospitals themselves, district nursing and health visiting, the blood transfusion service, occupational therapy and family planning services, although there are many others. The term 'voluntary organisation' covers those non-profit-making associations of individuals (or organisations) which are not created by statute. Depending on their constitution or statement of objects, they may be registered charities, registered companies, chartered bodies or have some other legal status. The contribution of voluntary organisations alongside the statutory provision of health and social services is considerable. Governments continue to recognise that this cooperation is mutually beneficial since in some cases the work of the voluntary organisations supplements that provided by the State (or vice versa), while in other cases the voluntary organisations fill in the gaps of State provision. There is, however, an important distinction between voluntary and statutory services.

Voluntary organisations often identify particular areas of need and specialise in educating public opinion on the deficiencies and potential improvements in statutory services, and they can often do this more flexibly and experimentally than a statutorily prescribed organisation.

Those organisations registered under the Charities Act 1960 (probably the majority in the health and welfare area) enjoy a number of financial benefits. Much of their income is derived from donations, legacies, government grants and fund-raising activities. They are entitled to direct relief of tax payable on this as well as being able to reclaim the tax paid by individuals on donations given as a covenant, and being allowed considerable relief on the rates payable on their premises. Some of the larger charities also derive a part of their income from their capital assets. Money is required to cover staff wages and administrative costs, advertising campaigns, research support and direct grants. The increasing inflation of recent years has put considerable financial pressure on many charities, particularly those whose income from year to year is less predictable. *Care in Action* encouraged the use of voluntary organisations as agents of the health authorities, because they could be more sensitive to new demands. Many existing voluntary bodies could not exist however without money from health and local authorities. The voluntary and statutory services are mutually dependent.

The contribution of the voluntary sector has become more controversial in the 1980s. To mark the beginning of the decade, circular HC(80)11[6] encouraged health authorities to involve themselves in fund raising if this seemed beneficial: previously direct fund raising had not been allowed. In the discussions leading up to the 1982 reorganisation, the then Secretary of State, Patrick Jenkin, suggested that much more could be provided by the voluntary sector leaving the statutory bodies as a 'safety net' to ensure no-one was left without support.[7] Such a view was an anathema to the Labour party, in Opposition at the time. Even less acceptable was the idea that voluntary work was a suitable alternative for paid work at times of unemployment. Indeed, despite a sharp rise in unemployment, volunteers were not always easy to recruit. Health services have long been supported by leagues of hospital friends and numerous other bodies but it seems unlikely that large sums of money can be raised on a recurring basis to become a realistic alternative to central funding.

Voluntary bodies and CHCs are not the only way the public can influence the NHS. Pressure groups, particularly those set up with a specific purpose, such as the saving of a hospital from closure have had several successes. The media, newspapers, radio and television, have become increasingly interested in health matters, particularly those related to high technology medicine and to hospital life. Informed radio and television programmes involve the public in medical research and new treatments. Even popular fiction as represented by a television series should not be discounted. A recent series called *Angels* has covered many areas of concern from how best to care for the elderly to epilepsy and solvent abuse. The media thrive on hospital closure stories and contributed to the success of both the Elizabeth Garrett Anderson Hospital and Tadworth Court campaigns.[8] In the former case, the hospital, one of the two remaining hospitals run by women for women, was kept open. Ironically the outcome of this case, which involved the health authority concerned in numerous practical problems because of the poor condition of the building, may have contributed to the failure of a similar campaign to preserve the South London Hospital for Women, which closed despite opposition some three years later. Tadworth Court, the country branch of the Children's Hospital of Great Ormond Street, London, was handed over to the voluntary sector with a considerable subsidy.

Since the first reorganisation, health authorities and their staff have become more responsive to their role as agents of the public they serve and a more open attitude to the media has resulted. The media, in their turn, can do much to protect the rights of the public. This is particularly important in matters of research and to ensure patients are not abused in other ways.

Medical Research and Intervention

Research into new and more effective forms of treatment is a necessary and expected activity, and the benefits of its results are well known. However, a strong body of opinion is opposed to certain techniques and experiments both on animal and human subjects. The State finances research directly through the Medical Research Council and through grants to individuals, and indirectly through its funding of academic institutions which carry out research, and most of this work is carefully done. Concern has arisen over cases where the rights of the subjects may appear to have been disregarded. In 1967, Dr M.H. Papp-worth published a book called *Human Guinea Pigs*[9] in which he documented over seventy experiments using human subjects in Britain which were dangerous, unethical and, sometimes, illegal. The response of some members of the medical profession was embarrassed and defensive, but a direct result was the establishment of committees of doctors in hospitals to vet all new proposals for clinical research. This acknowledged that the responsibility for deciding on the ethics of an experiment should not rest with the investigator alone, and by 1975 the DHSS issued a circular advising that lay members, possibly from community health councils, should join these ethical committees.[10]

In the case of developing new drugs, the Medicines Commission scrutinises methods of testing, but it still remains true that animal and human subjects have to be used at an early stage, before a medicine can be known to be safe and effective or not. The case of thalidomide illustrates a possible outcome of insufficient preparatory research. The drug thalidomide was first synthesised in Germany in 1956 and marketed as a sedative and hypnotic. In 1958 it became manufactured and marketed in Britain under licence to Distillers Company Biochemicals Ltd, under several brand names including 'Distaval'. It was found to be a particularly effective sedative which did not have some disadvantages of the barbiturates, and was prescribed for pregnant women to reduce feelings of tension. In November 1961 a German paediatrician reported the suspected connection between congenital deformities in babies and the use of thalidomide in early pregnancy. On 2 December 1961 Distillers announced withdrawal of the drug. About 8,000 deformed children were born as a result of the use of thalidomide, over 400 of them in Britain.[11] Legal actions against Distillers have been pursued by a number of the children and settlements have been made in other cases, some following an investigation by Sir Alan Marre, largely completed in 1978.

This affair was one of the factors contributing to the revised legislation on the testing of new drugs and the advertising of their properties. Even when drugs have been thoroughly developed, the doubts about their safety can remain, as for example with certain steroid preparations and the contraceptive pill.

Another related problem which concerns the ethics of medical intervention is that of keeping people alive by artificial means. When heart transplants were first performed in the 1960s they captured the interest of the press, but the success rate was relatively disappointing. The high cost of the procedure and the problems of finding suitable donors at the right time have tended to work against much development in this area. Kidney transplantation however is being much more actively pursued. Many people with chronic renal failure are kept alive by being attached to a kidney machine for intermittent dialysis, but the demand for treatment far exceeds the availability of resources. However, the transplant operation is technically less difficult than for the heart, and if a suitable donor can be found, and the considerable problems of tissue rejection managed, a patient with a transplant can recover to lead a fully active and normal life. The untreated disease is fatal, and life with a kidney machine is full of difficulties, so transplantation can offer the best solution for many sufferers. In 1972 the DHSS launched a public campaign to encourage people to decide to allow their kidneys to be used for transplantation if they died. Response to the campaign was disappointing, and although many hospitals were fully equipped to perform the operation (except for shortages of technical staff in some places) people with the disease are dying because there are insufficient donors.

However, the decision on whether to prolong a patient's life or not can be extremely difficult to make, especially when facilities for their continuing care are in short supply. The increasing incidence of degenerative and terminal illnesses in old people bears witness to considerable mastery over the infectious and damaging diseases, and the poor social conditions that limited the life expectancy of earlier generations, but this brings problems with it. One observer has written: 'It is clearly pointless to keep a patient with an inoperable brain tumour breathing when a fatal outcome is certain, and in the case of recurrent chest infections in the elderly respiratory cripple there may come a time when it is unkind to rescue the patient yet again from an acute episode only to restore him to distressing permanent disablement. The decision to submit a patient to resuscitation or intensive therapy must be informed, deliberate and responsible'.[12] Cases of serious and possibly irreversible brain damage following road accidents or the birth of babies with congenital abnormalities such as spina bifida exercise the judgement of doctors and families to the extreme, and the definition of meaningful survival and the cost of intervention, both financial and emotional, have to be made somehow.

Matters raised in this chapter lead to the question: is the NHS yet sensitive enough to the public it serves? Health authorities themselves, the CHCs, voluntary bodies, pressure groups and the media all help to protect the public interest. Unlike some countries, litigation in the UK is not a significant factor in bringing about changes, because there is so little of it. In the early 1980s, the government took the view that more competition might improve standards and private hospitals were able to develop more rapidly. But the private sector still provides a very small part of patient care. Such provision did draw to health authorities' attention the somewhat scant concern most DHAs have for matters such as waiting time in outpatient departments, attitudes of staff, and the bigger issue of waiting lists. Opinion polls and other research have shown that the NHS remains a popular part of the welfare state. But recurrent scandals concerning long term care, the poor condition of many hospitals, and the waiting lists are still some of the hallmarks of the NHS which need to be tackled if the NHS intends to earn the continuing support of the majority of the public.

Notes

1. Department of Health and Social Security. *Democracy in the National Health Service*, HMSO, London, 1974.

2. DHSS Circular HC(80)8. *Health Service Development: Structure and Management*, July 1980.

3. DHSS Circular HC(81)15. *Health Service Development: Community Health Councils*, December 1981.

4. Department of Health and Social Security, Welsh Office. *Report of the Committee on Hospital Complaints Procedure* (Chairman, Sir Michael Davies), HMSO, London, 1973.

5. DHSS, SHHD, Welsh Office. *Report on Operation of Procedure for Independent Review of Complaints involving the Clinical Judgement of Hospital Doctors and Dentists*, November, 1983.

6. DHSS Circular HC(80)11. *Health Service Management Health Services Act 1980: Fund Raising by NHS Authorities*, December 1980.

7. Patrick Jenkin, Article in *The Guardian*, 26 January, 1981.

8. Elizabeth Garrett Anderson Hospital is a Women's Hospital and became the centre of a purposeful campaign stimulated as much by the women's movement as by the desire to keep the hospital open for its own sake, particularly when the conditions were poor. The Prime Minister, Margeret Thatcher, publicly supported the campaign. Tadworth Court, an annexe to Great Ormond Street Hospital for sick children was reprieved by the Minister of State (Health) Kenneth Clarke and subsequently offered to the Spastics Society to run. The continuing financial difficulties suggested that the decision to stay open had little to do with financial sense but a great deal to do with political expediency.

9. M.H. Pappworth, *Human Guinea Pigs: Experimentation on Man*, Routledge and Kegan Paul, London, 1967.

10. Great Britain, Department of Health and Social Security. Welsh Office. Health Service Circular (Interim Series) HSC(IS)153, *Supervision of the Ethics of Clinical Research Investigations and Fetal Research*, DHSS, London, 1975.

11. Ministry of Health. Reports on Public Health and Medical Subjects No. 112. *Deformities caused by Thalidomide*, HMSO, London, 1964.

12. Henry Miller, *Medicine and Society*, Oxford University Press, London, 1973, p. 62.

It is claimed that the NHS provides the best value for money of all health care systems of the industrialised western countries. How true this is will be discussed here by comparing patients' access to health care, the quality of that care and how the various countries finance their health service.

Comparison with third-world countries is not really meaningful given that so much of the ill-health there is due to infectious diseases. The work of the World Health Organisation has been significant in reducing and, in the case of smallpox, eliminating infectious diseases, but poor water supplies remain the most significant source of disease in many countries. Some states, especially those which have become rich from oil revenues during the last 20 years, have superimposed western-style hospitals on a relatively underdeveloped society. Where this prosperity subsequently collapses, as in Nigeria, the sophisticated western-style medicine is likely to wane, exposing the public health problems again. The USSR offers an interesting bridge between the sophistication of industrialised countries and the basic problems still being tackled by the third-world. Although much has been done the control of infectious diseases in many parts of the USSR still lags behind.

Access to Health Care

People's ability to obtain health care is determined by three factors: social or racial standing, financial status and where they live. First, social or racial standing. As has been stated, the Black report[1] established that people in the UK belonging to lower occupational classes suffer more ill-health. The evidence suggests that if the mortality rates of class I (professional people and their families) were applied to classes IV and V (manual workers and their families) during 1970–72, as many as 74,000 lives would not have been prematurely lost. The reasons for this are largely outside the control of the health service and include low income, poor housing, less education, and consequently a comparatively deprived lifestyle. How far are these findings applicable in other countries? The Black report wrestled with the inherent difficulties of making international comparisons[2] where the statistics do not have a common base, but nevertheless concluded in its study of infant mortality that socio-economic factors were usually influential, although differences between countries stimulated more questions than answers. It is not clear why the results are so much better in Sweden and Norway than in England. How has France improved its position so markedly in a relatively short period?

In the UK the NHS is available to all irrespective of their social class. Some other countries demonstrate more class-related services. In the USA middle-class people widely use private sources of care based on a fee for services system. But poor people, those living in inner cities and racial minority groups have to rely on a public system, mostly based on the local county or city hospital. Unlike the middle-class middle-income patients who have potentially limitless choice, the disadvantaged have little choice. West Germany has a tiered hospital system in which paying more money buys a better level of service and access to more experienced and senior doctors. The pre-selection of patients has much in common with pre-1948 Britain where access to the voluntary hospital often required a member of the management board to sponsor them, while patients could be admitted to municipal hospitals directly.

A fundamental principle of the NHS was that patients should be treated equally, entirely irrespective of their financial means. Despite the increase in private medicine which allows people to buy themselves prompt treatment instead of having to queue on the waiting list, this principle has remained largely intact. But there still remains a hidden discriminator. Studies have shown that middle-class people use the NHS more, as well as more effectively, than the working class do. This is true in the preventive field where screening programmes, for instance cervical cytology, often fail to reach those women most at risk. High socio-economic status is associated with more knowledgeable patients who are more able to make better use of the services available. In other countries the same effect is observed. In the USA those with money can afford as much health care as they like, those without have limited choice, but are also restricted to more heavily controlled services where even the number of consultations or referrals to hospitals are regulated.

The Royal Commission undertook a study to check whether location within the UK was significant in influencing access to health care.[3] This study looked at a rural community in Cumbria and a London borough, and found that patients in both these places were satisfied with their access to care, at least at the primary level. The public support for retaining local hospitals in the UK suggests that physical proximity is an important consideration. But how do other countries manage where distances are much greater? Sweden is a country with a population of only 8.2 million of which 3 million live in three cities, yet the remainder are spread thinly over an area bigger than Italy, Austria and Switzerland combined. As in Canada, health facilities in Sweden have to be widely spaced. In France, legislation in 1958–68 developed a three-tiered system of university hospitals, general hospitals and local hospitals. The USSR has a system of regional hospitals, town hospitals, district hospitals and sector hospitals, although this last group are very small and not always covered by medical staff. Other countries such as Germany, the Netherlands and the USA have a less organised system, but by using planning regulations they are attempting to rationalise hospital provision and reduce maldistribution. The actual distribution of hospitals tends to be determined by the population distribution characteristics of that country. In the United Kingdom, 10 miles may be seen as being too far from the nearest hospital, while in rural Sweden 100 miles might be considered reasonable.

Does distance from a hospital lead to poorer levels of health care? Apparently not. Sweden achieves some of the best results in the world with, for instance, an infant mortality rate at way below the UK's present figure of 11 (1982). Furthermore, the most remote county in Sweden has the lowest rate in Sweden itself. Distance is not necessarily significant in itself, but the type of physical environment plainly is. Industrial urban areas are more polluted than rural areas and there is a price to pay for that in health terms. During the 1970s the EEC introduced action programmes aimed at reducing pollution by waste, chemicals and noise. Food poisoning has become a significant international hazard.

The variations in access to health care which relate to class, financial and geographical factors are important, but equally significant is the actual availability of health care provision: there is little point in seeking health care if there are no doctors or other health care workers and no hospitals or clinics. The policies controlling distribution of these facilities is therefore crucial. There are marked differences between western countries. Access to treatment is largely determined by doctors. One of the successes of the NHS is that the distribution of family doctors is now much more even than before. GPs have an average of around 2,200 patients on their lists and because of the system of regulation (see Chapter 8) the number of doctors working in each area is controlled. In West Germany a system of incentives was introduced in 1976 to encourage doctors to practise in unpopular areas, but these were not general practitioners in the English sense. Indeed, only Denmark and the Netherlands have a system of general practice remotely comparable to the English system. In other countries, there is no difference between general practitioners and hospital doctors. A doctor will first see a patient in his own surgery and then if the patient needs hospital care, will take him into hospital or refer him to a colleague. Outpatient departments are not found in some countries. In West Germany outpatient departments have only recently been established and then only in university hospitals. In Sweden, community health centres covering a population of between 20,000 and 50,000 provide both primary care and outpatient consultation. In Norway, with smaller health centres, the outpatient element is less significant. In the USSR there are an estimated 36,000 polyclinics. Since 1947 it has been policy to unify them with hospitals in urban areas in order to improve standards. By 1970 about 75 per cent of polyclincs were attached to a hospital of some type. This in turn has apparently caused some problems of access due to distance.

The most common system, found in Germany, USA, France and other countries, allows patients to attend specialist doctors' own surgeries of their choice or in some cases as referred by their employer. The doctor then decides how best to deal with the patient. This system is under considerable criticism in these countries and has several disadvantages. First, patients may make the wrong choice and consequently be at risk from inappropriate treatment from a specialist not well informed in the appropriate specialty. Secondly, their care will be uncoordinated and treatment for single episodes of illness tends overall to be less suitable. Thirdly, this can lead to waste as the more affluent patients may go to more than one doctor for the same complaint. In West Germany and Sweden, where the number of hospital beds per population is generous, patients may be admitted to hospital unnecessarily.

The total number of doctors affect the situation too and there are wide variations; West Germany and Sweden are well provided with one doctor for approximately 450 and 600 members of the population respectively. The USA has about 770, but this disguises major variations between heavily populated cities at around 1 doctor per 500 and remote rural areas with a figure 1 to 2,500. England and Wales and France have roughly similar numbers of about 1 per 1,000 population. In France, however, maldistribution is a problem the government has been trying to tackle. 35,000 of the 46,000 doctors are private practitioners and the regulation of these has brought about major conflicts with the government.

Doctors are paid differently from country to country. In the Netherlands there is increasing pressure to employ doctors on a direct salary. As in Sweden where 85 per cent of doctors are publicly employed, this seems likely to gain support even from doctors themselves because it would eradicate major differences in earning power between doctors. In this respect, Sweden is the most radical of all western countries where fees were abolished in 1959 for hospital care and in 1970 for ambulatory (outpatient or community) care. In the NHS, the original NHS Act and the 1966 GP Charter moved the other way as a perceived political trade-off for developing general practice primary care. In the late 1970s, hospital doctors endeavoured to improve their contracts in a similar way, but the basis of their payment system has not yet been substantially changed.

In the countries mentioned, the number of doctors has increased and often doubled in the last 30 years to the point where some countries feel that they have too many doctors. In the NHS entry to medical schools has been pegged, but even so there are said to be about 1000 unemployed doctors. Recent regulation of medical school intake in France has been unpopular. In the USA, as in the UK, regulation of medical schools started in 1910. Current estimates suggest that the country as a whole is becoming over-doctored, but local distribution varies widely.

The work of doctors is not only determined by the needs and demands of their patients, but also the availability of hospital beds and other facilities. In the UK a shortage of beds is often cited as the reason for long waiting lists. The occupancy of beds allocated to acute care is poor, since roughly a quarter of them are empty at any one time. The USA and other countries which rely on a payment system for occupied beds per day have a vested interest in maximising the use of beds and their management tends to be affected by these considerations. Whether the patient needs to be in the bed is another question. We know that operation rates between England and the USA vary widely and some surgical procedures are being undertaken in the USA much more frequently than here. Continential European countries also have a higher level of bed provision than the UK. The Netherlands has about 5.5 beds per 1,000 population for short-term care (comparable to what the UK calls acute), West Germany has 7.7 beds, and DHSS guidance allows only 2.8. In Sweden the allocation of beds for the elderly is said to be eight times that allowed in England (now running here at between 8.5 and 10 per 1,000 population over sixty-five). Admissions to these beds have increased in all countries at the same time as the length of stay has shortened. Despite this, there are still wide discrepancies which are difficult to account for.

It is difficult to draw conclusions regarding a 'correct' number of beds. Influential factors are the extent of community and primary care, the availability of outpatient facilities, the extent of market competition between hospitals and the historical supply of beds.

Finally, the number of beds has a major effect on the cost of the service so that the relatively low level of total allocation to the NHS as reflected in the proportion of the GNP is not surprising given the relatively low number of beds. Most other countries are worried about the high cost of hospital services and acknowledge that they have too many beds or that these tend to be wastefully used. To a certain extent this is due to the way doctors exercise control over hospital resources.

Clinical autonomy (or liberalism as it is sometimes called in other countries) allows doctors to make decisions about patient care free of cost considerations. In Sweden, fees for service have been largely eliminated. In England, what doctors may charge is regularised in the public sector although not in the small private sector. In the Netherlands recent legislation is changing over from a fee-for-service to a salaried arrangement for hospital doctors. GPs there are paid on the number of patients registered with them. In the USA various attempts are being made to reduce the increasing level of doctors' fees for instance by Health Maintenance Organizations which were introduced in 1973, enabling doctors to set up pre-paid group practice systems. In this way they have become able to provide a more comprehensive level of care with less reliance on hospitals and at correspondingly lower cost.

Quality of Service

Countries vary in their attempts to control the quality of service which doctors provide. The NHS has lagged behind in this respect. It is a public service under the scrutiny of health authorities within the governing framework, but the attempts at quality control have been limited to advisory systems such as the Health Advisory Service, the Development Team for the Handicapped and Community Health Councils. What is missing is the systematic review of clinical performance in the acute sector, although with the emerging interest in performance indicators, a change may be occurring. Medical audit is seldom found in the UK except where individual consultants have shown a particular interest. There is no official system of audit. The Royal Colleges, however, can exert some sanctions where they judge standards are too low, by withholding recognition of junior doctor posts for training. General practitioners are subject only to mild scrutiny on their drug prescribing. It is ironic that in a service which is run by the State, so little control of the standards of performance and the quality of care have been established.

Other countries have done more. Although health services in the USA are apparently allowed to flourish in the open market of free enterprise they are in fact heavily regulated. All doctors have to be licensed practitioners, but beyond this there is a system for further professional accreditation after post-graduate training. Hospitals themselves are also exposed to accreditation procedures. The Joint Commission on the Accreditation of Hospitals (JCAH) assesses hospitals every two years on their organisational structure, physical environment and the staffing levels. More recently JCAH has started to examine medical audits undertaken within hospitals by their own staff. Hospitals carry out the accreditation voluntarily, but those failing to meet the standards set face the withdrawal of federal or state funds and a consequent loss of financial viability. In 1972 the US Department of Health Education and Welfare set up the Professional Standards Review Organization (PSRO). One hundred and ninety-five PSROs undertake reviews of utilisation of facilities which are partly stimulated by the rising cost of the Medicare and Medicaid federally funded systems (discussed below). These reviews are undertaken by physicians themselves, but examine individual medical practice in detail. PSROs have been unpopular and some critics doubt whether they have materially controlled the inflation in hospital costs.[4]

France has a well articulated system of inspection. About 4,000 physicians employed by the social security administration have to authorise costly procedures and scrutinise lengthy stays in hospital. The system is bureaucratic and resented, but the inspectors are well paid and there is no difficulty in recruitment. Hospitals themselves are inspected by a smaller body of civil servants at Department level. At national level a further body, usually staffed by administrators, undertakes special studies and issues an annual report. There are also groups of auditors who have the right to examine any aspect of the country's administration. Recent reports from them have drawn attention to poor standards in some French hospitals.

Financial Control

A major concern of all governments is to control the cost of health care. All countries mentioned here have that problem, despite their different methods of financing health care. The Secretary of State in 1982/83 is understood to have reviewed the various systems for financing health care. After some interest in switching to an insurance based scheme he concluded that the present method largely dependent on direct taxation (see Chapter 6) was probably better than any other. Certainly the British system is simpler than others and this is reflected in the lower administrative costs of the service. It is said that administrative costs in the USA are over 20 per cent, in France 10 per cent, but in the United Kingdom less than 5 per cent.

Although Sweden and England have a State-financed system, the Swedish health service allows for twenty-three county councils and three county boroughs to raise 75 per cent of the total finance through local taxation. Recently there has been a move towards greater central control, particularly vetting new capital buildings and manpower developments. The federation of county councils negotiates with the National Board of Health and Welfare. From the 1960s the high standard of living and relative equality in modern Sweden led to an explosion in health care facilities and expenditure, but more recently a flattening of economic growth rates has required the costs to be controlled more rigorously. In common with other countries, the number of elderly in Sweden has increased and so have the demands for high technology medicine.

The system in the Netherlands is markedly different from the NHS, in that a large proportion of health care is provided by the private sector, but controlled through a series of Acts of Parliament, such as the two Hospital Facilities Acts of 1972 and 1979 and the even more recent Health Services Act 1984. Private fees account for 25 per cent of the total budget of health care and the rest comes from the Sickness Fund Insurance Scheme set up in 1964 (43 per cent) the Special Sickness Expenses provisions (27 per cent) and a small proportion of direct state funding. The West German system is acknowledged to be complicated. Insurance covers over 90 per cent of the population of whom 57 per cent are compulsorily insured, 13 per cent voluntarily insured and 30 per cent retired but insured. State employees get between 50 per cent and 70 per cent refund for services received, but many take out private insurance to cover the cost not reimbursed by the State. Regulations under the 1972 and 1982 Hospitals Laws have attempted to control expenditure through more coherent planning. The Cost Control Law of 1977 aimed to reduce expenditure and also introduced cost sharing mechanisms such as direct charges to patients for dentures and for spa treatment (a form of care somewhat derided in the NHS).

Under the French system, patients pay in full first and then claim back roughly 75 per cent of the cost. Within that, 80 per cent of inpatient costs are charged direct to the patient's insurance fund leaving the remainder to be met by the patient. The system is currently under review (1984). The costs themselves vary geographically and are related to doctors' fees. But insurance cover is by no means universal and in the early 1970s it was estimated that 80 per cent of the population under the age of 35 were covered, but of the over 80s only 51 per cent of men and 29 per cent of women were covered. A social aid programme therefore exists to support those not covered and those suffering from chronic illness, such as TB or mental disorder.

In the USA the system is most confusing. Broadly speaking, health care is financed in four different ways. First, from private practice on a fee-for-service basis; secondly, by local government particularly for the poor inner city and minority groups; thirdly, through the Veterans Administration system and fourthly by the military authorities. Only the last of these could be said to be well organised and integrated, because the scope extends only to a finite population and the organisation is susceptible to clear procedures. The Veterans Administration is predominantly a hospital service and looks after retired and disabled people who previously served in the forces. It is therefore largely for men. It is exposed to considerable consumer and political pressure. The local government programme is heavily supported by federal funds in the form of Medicaid set up in 1965 to provide a safety net for those too poor to be eligible for private health care insurance schemes. Medicare is also funded by federal government and provides cover for all people over 65. County and city hospitals, private hospitals and many nursing homes recover the daily cost of patients they treat under these two schemes. The system allows the standards of these institutions to be scrutinised and if they are found unsatisfactory funds may be withdrawn. For instance, a South Carolina hospital slow to integrate black and white patients was threatened with the withdrawal of federal funds, which, if implemented would have closed the hospital; integration therefore took place.[5]

Private practice in the USA is available for anyone capable of paying or who has an insurance company ready to do so. The heavy reliance on this system has inflated health care cost so that by 1980 9.4 of the GNP was being spent on health care in the USA and yet the services remained ill coordinated and underplanned. This is despite the National Health Planning and Resources Development Act, which in 1974 had provided a major impetus to plans to cut some of the waste inherent in the multiplicity of health care systems. Up to the mid-1960s, government funds contributed only about 25 per cent of the total health care budget, but by 1975 this had increased to 43 per cent. The Reagan administration in the early 1980s became increasingly unhappy with this commitment and endeavoured to shift expenditure from federal government to the states and to encourage more cost sharing with the consumer, whilst preserving a basic minimum level of service. For the poor inner city dweller the minimum standard may be very low indeed for a highly developed country.

The financing of health care is a problem to all these countries. All governments find themselves spending more than they wish, all complain of waste and poor control, all are worried for the future. Significantly, all the countries have introduced major legislation in the last ten years to attempt to control costs and financial allocations. It seems that whatever the ideological stance of the government, more state involvement in control is inevitable. Will this also be true for the NHS? The increasing interest in cost-sharing through privatisation, the developing interest in the use of performance indicators and the determination to have a more accountable management all echo the concern of other countries and their governments. 'Socialised medicine', much feared by some of these countries, together with the persistent problem of waiting lists, may in turn become characteristic of other systems as well as the UK's. Despite the problems facing the NHS, the service received for the resources provided still makes it relatively cost effective in comparison with similar countries elsewhere in the western world.

Notes

1. DHSS. *Report of the Working Group on Inequalities in Health* (Black Report), HMSO, London, 1980.

2. This chapter faces the same difficulties, but the literature of international comparisons is expanding. Useful books are McLachlan and Maynard, *The Public/Private Mix for Health*, Nuffield Provincial Hospitals Trust, London, 1982; Robert Maxwell, *Health Care: the Growing Dilemma*, 2nd edn., McKinsey & Co., 1976

and *Health and Wealth: an International Study of Health-care Spending*, Clexington Books, 1981; Miziahi, Mizrahi and Sandier *Medical Care, Mobility and Costs*, Pergamon, Oxford, 1983.

3. Simpson, R. *Access to Primary Care*, Research Paper No. 6, Royal Commission on the National Health Service, HMSO, London, 1978.

4. For an account of PSROs see Williams and Towers, *Introduction to Health Services*, John Wiley & Son, New York, 1980, pp. 345–346.

5. For a full account of this see: Hepner, James O. (ed.), *Hospital Administrator – Physician Relationships*, C.V. Mosby, St. Louis, 1980.

14 THE NHS AND THE FUTURE

The NHS is one of the largest employers in the world with a staff of nearly a million people. For this reason alone it will remain a matter of consuming interest for any British government. To work well it needs stability, but it must equally be responsive to changes in need and to economic fluctuations. This chapter discusses some of the main issues facing the NHS and attempts to explore how these will change over the next few years. First, the chapter looks at the pattern of need and demand. Then there is a discussion on resources and finally an examination of the options for organising the supply of health care.

Need and Demand

Need and demand are interrelated, but are not the same. Need is based on an objective assessment against known criteria. For instance, given that the very old have more ill-health than the rest of the population, what services are needed by them? Demand, on the other hand, is more volatile and is based on the expectations, realistic or not, of the population. Heart transplants, operations of considerable cost with a relatively unproven success rate, nevertheless catch the public imagination and are widely supported. Managers of the health service are left with the task of reconciling needs and demands knowing that resources are not always available to satisfy both.

The Royal Commission at the beginning of its task tried to satisfy all opinion by listing the objectives of the NHS:

Figure 32 *Objectives of the NHS*

    Encourage and assist individuals to remain healthy
    Provide equality of entitlement to health services
    Provide a broad range of services of high standard
    Provide equality of access to these services
    Provide a service free at the time of use
    Satisfy the reasonable expectations of its users
    Remain a national service responsive to local needs

Source: Royal Commission on the NHS, 1979

This was in effect a manifesto for the NHS but was by no means satisfied in 1979, the year of the Royal Commission's report, or indeed since. This fact was of course recognised by the Royal Commission itself when it said later in its report 'the NHS reflects the society around it — both society's aspirations towards good health and its careless attitudes towards bad health'.[2] Surveys have shown that very few people, when asked how they felt during the last fortnight, responded that they had been completely well. Many had had symptoms which whilst not requiring the attendance at a doctors' surgery or hospital, had needed some sort of treatment. The demand for health services is potentially limitless. If a long-term cure for headaches could be found, people at present prescribing themselves aspirin would no doubt go to their doctor to get on the waiting list for the cure. Such an example may seem unrealistic until it is realised that joint replacement, one of the main contributors to hospital waiting lists, was not a viable operation until well after the start of the NHS. Before that time patients had to endure their arthritis as best they could. Demand and need cannot be separated. Patients who know that their pain and incapacity can be relieved will naturally demand the operation, but as most of these patients are elderly and because their disability makes them reliant on the services of the district nurse, the community occupational therapist, social workers, the meals on wheels service, they clearly have a genuine need. Health service planners have to work out the likely need before they plan what services to provide. It is known that the rise in the percentage of elderly during the next fifteen years will be considerable. In 1976 1 in 104 of hospital inpatients was 85 years old or over, but by the end of the century this will have increased to 1 in 64. There are twice as many women over 75 as men. Despite these figures only about six per cent of people over the age of 65 live in residential or hospital accommodation. The options for the future depend upon policy decisions as to the level of sheltered and residential care compared with support at home. Despite considerable discussion, health authorities and the government in the early 1980s had made little coherent preparation for this increase in need.

One of the reasons for the inadequate provision of services for the elderly or indeed other disadvantaged groups such as the mentally ill or the mentally handicapped, has been the well articulated demands of the acute sector of care which can loosely be described as those services provided by district general hospitals. These hospitals have always taken the largest proportion of resources and have been better staffed and better equipped than other hospitals. To date relatively little work has been done to prove the effectiveness of many of the medical procedures undertaken in acute hospitals. In 1972 A.L. Cochrane pointed out[3] that the effectiveness of many of these procedures was totally untested, even when it would have been possible to set up what he called randomised controlled trials. More recent research has shown that the results of the majority of laboratory and radiological tests and examinations do not lead to changes in patients' treatment. The Royal Commission stressed the point calling medicine 'an inexact science'. This dilemma cannot be resolved. If doctors were only to do what they know to be effective, medical science would stagnate. Experimentation is often necessary to establish what will be good for a patient.

Each year the DHSS's chief Medical Officer of Health produces a report *On the State of Public Health*.[4] This reviews the work of the past year and indicates those aspects of treatment which are likely to make new demands on the NHS. The 1981 report listed the following: a new method of treatment for chronic kidney failure; coronary by-pass grafting; improved pacemaker technology for patients suffering from heart disease; further development in fibre optics used to view internal organs without the need for surgery; the development of parenteral nutrition (a method of feeding through the bloodstream for patients with bowel disease); the use of lasers to overcome blindness affecting some diabetic patients; further advances in joint replacement; developments in computerised tomography (CT scanning) which provides better information than most other forms of radiology and with less radiation to the patient. Many of these advances rely on high technology and as a result medical physics departments have continued to grow. Not all such developments prove their worth and doctors are as likely to be prone to temporary enthusiasms as any other professional group. The influence of professionals on demand is substantial. Most patients believe their doctor when he says that the treatment he is providing is in the patient's best interest; demand tends to be led by the professions rather than the patients themselves. This may lead to some distortion of priorities. Other NHS staff such as nurses and administrators may find that they have to provide a balancing force to correct these distortions by acting as advocates for the more disadvantaged groups whose needs are not met by medical technology.

Governments are not exempt from the influence professional pressure groups try to exert and special allocations to particular units show the success of those efforts. Nevertheless a government has the responsibility for ensuring that its policies meet the needs of the whole population. To respond to demands only would be highly inequitable and lead to large gaps in service provision. It seems likely that the present tension between high technology medicine on the one hand and increasing unmet need of disadvantaged groups on the other will continue to face the governments of the next decade.

What is meant by a disadvantaged group? They have been categorised into three groups, those disadvantaged by where they live, those disadvantaged by their social class and thirdly those disadvantaged by their medical condition. In the discussion on RAWP[5] in Chapter 6, it was shown that the allocation of resources was unequal and that the London Regions received more than others. The Black report on Inequalities[6] produced a detailed description of social inequality and showed that ill-health increased with lower occupational class so that a manual worker and his family could expect more illness than a professional man and his family. These findings pose important questions as to whether there should be positive discrimination in favour of lower occupational class groups. If this were done it would go further than the RAWP recommendations which were based largely on the assumption that it would be fair to give equal resources to all Regions irrespective of social need, although the formula did allow some adjustments for factors such as age distribution and mortality rates. Government response to the Black report was cool because the resource implications were too substantial. In the last decade government policy has acknowledged the need to reduce client group inequalities. Chapter 7 gave a detailed account of developments in the care of these groups and showed how, for instance, government policy underwritten by earmarked financial allocations had tried to improve the lot of groups such as the mentally handicapped. Despite recurrent scandals, it is doubtful whether public opinion alone would have insisted upon action, and therefore to improve services, an official acknowledgement of need was necessary. It had been said, however, that governments are more concerned to appear to respond to needs than to do so in reality. This argument is not grounded in cynicism so much as in a view of government, which holds that governments are there to satisfy the electors rather than change the society — governments are therefore largely symbolic in function. This interpretation ignores the strength of pressure groups, particularly those working as advocates of certain client groups. It seems likely that these will become stronger and following the experience in the USA, may increasingly turn to the processes of law to secure clients' rights. Anti-discrimination legislation has become a more prominent feature in the last decade providing additional opportunities to protect clients' and patients' status. How much can be done to support these groups and the demands excited by the development of medical technology depends largely on the resources that can be made available.

The Resource Problem

The NHS is largely financed from general taxation with national insurance contributions and other charges contributing scarcely more than 10 per cent to the overall budget. The NHS, therefore, is inextricably linked with the state of the economy. Chapter 6 showed that the proportion of the gross national product (GNP) spent on the NHS was less than most other industrialised countries, but that despite this value for money was probably good, at least in so far as all citizens had reasonable access to treatment and care. Successive governments have had to face the problem of increasing demand and, as in the case of the elderly, increasing need. Where can the money come from? Governments can still make small changes in allocations which are modest in monetary value yet substantial in their effect. Most arguments about funding in the NHS over recent years have been about very small percentage increases or decreases such that a health authority would consider itself well off if given 1.5 per cent increase for developments once inflation and pay awards have been met. From a government's point of view, an increase in charges for prescriptions or appliances has been worth the unpopularity.

It seems likely that the 1983 privatisation proposals will continue to be encouraged because even though the overall savings for each health authority are small, their impact could be considerable, at least in the short term. It will only be possible to judge in time whether the effect of privatisation has been inflationary. The present policy approach rests on the assumption that the NHS organisation of ancillary services is inefficient and that private contractors can do better, but if that proves to be wrong the financial benefits will be lost. The use of contractors in some services has already shown that the cost is not necessarily lower. Many parts of the country are unable to provide adequate chiropody services because chiropodists, who are able to treat self-referred patients, will not agree to change their contractual status to become directly employed. By doing this they would reduce their earning power. There is no reason, therefore, to assume that extending privatisation to cover many other services such as works, aspects of administration, and even some nursing and treatment facilities, will be a final answer to the NHS's financial problems.

If a government were to pursue the Jenkin 'safety-net'[7] principle whereby government protects people from destitution, but other agencies provide the services above that basic level, the NHS would be considerably diminished. The contracting out of most long stay accommodation and predictable acute care procedures such as operations for hernias or hip replacements, would lead to a system more like the French health system, where patients pay first and claim back afterwards. The danger of inflation is, however, always present. First, patients knowing that they were insured might be tempted to claim treatment whether they needed it or not. Secondly, the cost of administration of this sort of system is, as we have seen, considerable. Thirdly, insurance based schemes do nothing for those who are bad health risks or are too poor to pay premiums. As 60 per cent of patients are elderly, mentally ill, mentally handicapped or are children, the insurance solution, already in difficulties in other countries, appears to have little to offer. After some brief interest, the Conservative government of the early 1980s seemed to have accepted this fact.

It would appear, therefore, that alternative methods of funding the NHS are unlikely to flourish. If this is so, governments are left with increasing efficiency as the only realistic way of securing better services. In the 1970s, better planning was seen as the way in which resources could be more rationally used to the patients' best advantage. But many plans floundered because they were too ambitious and could not secure funds for their implementation. In the early 1980s the mood changed to be concerned with comparisons of performance. Auditors and others have demonstrated that there are many seeming anomalies up and down the country. Why should the cost of catering in hospital 'A' be twice that in hospital 'B', given that both have similar types of patients? If hospital 'B' can manage then so should hospital 'A' and funds would then be released for other use. Medical audit, never well received by the British medical profession, may increasingly be forced upon doctors so that cost and benefit accounts can be drawn up. In the wider area of resource management, the Ceri Davies report[8] on land use and management revealed substantial wasted assets which could be sold. This policy led to accusations that the government was only intent on asset stripping. Certainly the 1983 enthusiasm for manpower cuts was a way of freeing expenditure for other purposes. But what other purposes? The NHS is labour intensive with nearly 75 per cent of its funds spent on staff. With increasing technological sophistication on the one hand, but the dependence of increasing numbers of the very old on the other, it is difficult to see the proportion of staff falling substantially.

Rhetoric of successive government ministers fulminating against waste within the NHS will never disguise the inevitable political nature of resource allocation to health care. The NHS, despite its many shortcomings, is a popular service with the majority of people. Cuts in service are unwelcome as are increases in charges. The government, therefore, has to support the NHS and this was a keystone of the 1983 general election campaign.[9] But the limited resources must be efficiently allocated and used. Cash limits have made sure that authorities do not overspend. The percentage of the GNP devoted to health care may seem a matter of public debate, but the public are represented by health authorities who are required to show a degree of loyalty to the government of the day. How might future changes in the organisational structure safeguard or threaten this relationship?

Organisational Structure

It is perhaps inevitable that an organisation as big as the NHS should worry governments. Size suggests power, but also inflexibility. If all health authorities rebelled against a major policy decision, the government would find it difficult to insist. The matter of accountability has therefore become increasingly important since the first reorganisation in 1974. Governments wanted to ensure that their policies were implemented and the famous phrase 'maximum delegation downwards matched by maximum accountability upwards' was meant to resolve the dilemma as to how a government can insist on its policies being implemented whilst still allowing freedom of action by health authorities themselves. This issue is now much more prominent. The Conservative government elected in 1983 is pulling the reins of accountability tighter than before. Several notable tussles with health authorities since then have been won by the Secretary of State. The insistence on manpower cuts in the face of general opposition from health authorities demonstrated that accountability upwards had become much more important than delegation downwards. This was confirmed by the Griffiths report proposals which suggested a more authoritarian style of management that will replace the consensus style which had been the result of the 1974 reorganisation. The Griffiths report diagnosis that there was a want of leadership and consequently a lack of drive in the NHS reflected the government's perceptions. Increasing opposition to the proposals, not only from doctors and nurses, but also from some health authorities, may make further changes in the organisation of the NHS difficult to achieve. If this is so, and the government are unhappy with the outcome of the 1982 reorganisation, what other ways of organising the NHS remain?

As the Royal Commission pointed out, it had long been held in certain quarters that the NHS would be better run if it was part of local government. In this way the service would be more sensitive to local demand and because of the pressure of local democracy the influence of professionals would be somewhat reduced. The Royal Commission came to the conclusion that the NHS would not benefit from this move. In this they echoed the views expressed in the 1970 Green Paper, and they gave several reasons. First, as there was no regional tier in local government the task of the RHAs would have to be reallocated which would not be easy. Second, although strong arguments could be put forward that health and local authority services should be provided jointly, there was no reason to suppose that health would be better run by local government. This was not spelt out. Collaboration between health and local authority continues to be difficult in many places despite the inducements made available in the form of joint financing. Conterminosity of health and local authorities, abandoned as a guiding principle in the 1982 reorganisation, means that joint planning is more laborious. Prior to 1974, local authorities had run their own part of the NHS adequately. Third, the Royal Commission felt that to add health to local authorities would give too much work to one authority. Finally, it was felt that the considerable success of achieving a *national* health service with national standards would be lost if local authorities took over. This view was strongly held by others and an examination of the varying standards of local health authority provision would seem to support this view. The Royal Commission also examined the idea of a health commission or corporation which would give the NHS similar status to the BBC, the University Grants Committee or the Manpower Services Commission. It concluded that though there were some arguments in favour of such a change, the loss of accountability to Parliament was a serious impediment. Another way to run the NHS would be to contract out most of its services. As has been discussed above, such an arrangement might in the end be inflationary and would also make it even harder to maintain standards of care and treatment.

It seems therefore that the present system is likely to remain the most acceptable in that it provides reasonable safeguards for the public the NHS serves. If this reasoning is correct, health authorities will need to do much more to ensure that their role is not merely symbolic. The involvement of members in strategic planning is as much a responsibility as the more mundane duties of checking standards of care. Equally, those who work in the NHS will have themselves to blame if they do not demonstrate their ability to improve performance and quality of services, and governments therefore impose standards upon them. The NHS is one of the greatest feats of social and political endeavour. But it has to change with the times if it is to continue to be valued for what it does rather than because of a nostalgia for what it once stood for. Even though the NHS is a large and cumbersome organisation it does not necessarily have to become inflexible. There are clearly marked avenues of progress which need to be travelled along. The only real obstacle is people's attitudes. Hopefully the next two decades will see the NHS regain its vigour and equip itself to perform the humane service it was designed for.

Notes

1. *Royal Commission on the National Health Service*, HMSO, London, 1979 (Cmnd. 7615), para. 2.6, p. 9.

2. Ibid., para. 22.7, p. 356.

3. A.L. Cochrane. *Effectiveness and Efficiency*, Nuffield Provincial Hospitals Trust, Oxford, 1972.

4. DHSS. *On the State of the Public Health*, HMSO, London, each year.

5. DHSS. *Sharing Resources for Health in England*, HMSO, London, 1976.

6. DHSS. *Report of the Working Group on Inequalities in Health* (Black report), HMSO, London, 1980.

7. Patrick Jenkin, then Secretary of State, suggested in an article in *The Guardian* on 26 January 1981 that the function of the State was to provide a minimum standard, or 'safety net', to protect people from destitution. Any improvement on this standard should not be the responsibility of the State. This thinking seemed to hark back to the principles behind the 1834 Poor Law Amendment Act.

8. DHSS. *Underused and Surplus Property in the National Health Service* (Ceri Davies Report), HSMO, London, 1983.

9. The slogan often repeated by the Conservative party, was 'The NHS is safe in our hands'.

INDEX